A Lump in the Road

A Memoir

Terri Enghofer

Blessings
Terri Enghofer

i

ISBN-10: 1490915540
ISBN-13: 978-1490915548

Dedicated to Pauline. My spirit sister.
My reason for writing.

Forward

I knew it was bad news when Mom set up a three-way call with my brother and me. Her biopsy confirmed she had breast cancer. We listened carefully as she pragmatically explained the situation. They caught it early. It was treatable. She walked us through the details, and my initial fear of the word cancer soon dissipated. By the time we said our goodbyes, two thoughts dominated my mind: Cancer sucks. Mom will beat it.

I was a junior at UW-Madison putting a safe 70-mile distance between Mom's cancer and me. When I'd call home, we'd talk about school, work, or whatever was new in my life. She didn't allow her cancer to dominate our time together. I don't know how she juggled the piles of paperwork, bills, doctor appointments, and daily trips to the hospital for radiation along with her already jam-packed life. But she did, and still had time for Karl and me. Mom was still Mom.

Life is full of challenges. All we can control is how to overcome them. Mom faced her challenge one day at a time. After seven months of "one-days" she beat her cancer. I knew she would.

Dialogue within the story is to the best of the author's recollection, and some conversations may have been modified to provide artistic clarity; however, all speakers' personalities are reflected truthfully. All medical professionals' names have been changed to respect their privacy. These changes do not alter the story's authenticity, as experienced by the author.

Table of Contents

PART 1

—

Blindsided

1

Chapter 1

A shadow. A shadow almost undetectable to the naked eye. Only the very skilled and trained individual could argue the shadow even existed. As faint and seemingly inconspicuous as it appeared to be, the shadow had significance. And it had a name: Microcalcification.

"See this?"

See what?

"This shadow was not on your mammogram image last year. This needs investigating."

Investigating? That tiny shadow with the long name needs investigating?

And so the ball began to roll. Another mammogram at a different facility, this time with a magnification of the image. A new set of radiologist's eyes. The same assessment, plus a little bit more. The ball was getting bigger, like a snowball when you nudge it down a hill.

"This shadow should not be ignored. A biopsy would tell us more."

No WAY! A biopsy? The tiny shadow with the long name needs to be biopsied? Biopsy means cancer,

*doesn't it? Maybe I should get a second opinion.
Biopsies cost a lot of money.*

Another appointment. More time off work. If
the second opinion was the same as the first, I'd go with
the biopsy. Honestly. Who knew a tiny shadow could
cause such havoc? Its long name must have had
something to do with why everyone was so concerned.

The second-opinion doc agreed. He gave the
tiny shadow the exact same name and said it would be
in my best interest to have a biopsy performed. I had to
hear it twice. The procedure had a name, too:
stereotactic needle biopsy. The snowball got bigger
every time another medical professional got involved.

At the risk of sounding like a moron, I had to
ask, "Biopsy means we're looking for cancer, right?"

The doc looked at me like I had three heads.

"There's no need to worry at this point. Yes, we
are testing for the presence of cancer cells within the
microcalcification in your right breast, but truly, there's
only a five to ten per cent chance cancer will be
present."

"I don't mean to sound argumentative, but
someone has to make up the five to ten per cent.
People are in those statistics. Women people. Like
me."

"Again, it's too early to say. We'd be
speculating. I'm sorry. I thought I explained that's
why it's best to have this area biopsied. Then we'll
know for certain whether cancer cells are present."

I held back the rest of what I wanted to say to
this evidently too-bothered-to-entertain-my-fears-or-
questions doctor. I'm a mother. I know attitude when I
hear it, and the doc was starting to use attitude with me.

My internal fire was starting to rise up from my gut, and I knew if I continued the conversation I'd be spitting flames. He was really ticking me off, but the last thing I wanted was to be removed from his office by Security. I ended up paying $167.50 for his arrogance.

Chapter 2

I scheduled the biopsy. More time off work.
How much time? A couple of hours? Half of a work
day? The glossy brochure describing the procedure
suggested that I go home afterward, put my feet up, and
relax.

Relax? Who writes these things?

The biopsy did not go flawlessly. While the
radiologist was extracting the tissue sample, the needle
broke some blood vessels in my breast, which
instantaneously triggered the growth of a dangerously
severe bruise called a hematoma. He was unable to
take the time to draw additional suspicious tissue, since
controlling the hematoma took priority. The battle just
started, and already I was sporting a bruised, swollen,
purple breast resembling an eggplant, which was
grossly disproportionate to its neighbor on the left, the
sweet pea.

Nice going. These are professionals, right?

The radiology technician and a nurse packed me
with ice, wrapped me up tight like a sausage in a
casing, and urged me to go home . . . and relax. I did
go home, but I did not relax.

In the world that exists outside of glossy brochures, you do not relax after a biopsy. You panic. Your voice shakes, you gulp dry tension, and you eat, sleep, and shower with one hand on the telephone waiting for someone, anyone, to call you with the news that everything's all right. That phone call came the following day while I was at work. The voice on the other end of the phone asked me to come to the hospital to learn the results of my test. For whatever reason, this news couldn't be shared through the modern convenience of a telephone. I was pretty sure I knew the reason.

Should I stop relaxing? No problem. I never started.

I left the office around 2:00 and told my boss, Helen, I'd be back within the hour. It was a 15-minute drive to the hospital, and my heart raced with fear as possible scenarios rattled through my head. I nearly ran a red light when I felt a hand on my shoulder and heard the words, *"It's cancer, Terri. Get your affairs in order,"* whispered into my ear. By the time I pulled into the parking lot I could hardly let go of the steering wheel. I stared into my rearview mirror, afraid to look but more afraid to look away. The backseat was empty, but I could still feel the weight of that hand on my shoulder.

Stay calm. It's probably nothing. They probably botched the test and want to take more samples. I'm stressing over nothing.

The radiologist I thought I'd be meeting with was nowhere to be seen. I was ushered into a softly lit room, and 413 hours later a young, woman doctor in a crisp white lab coat floated into the room and sat down beside me. Before she uttered a single word, I knew by the ten-degree tilt of her head and raised eyebrows that she was not going to tell me everything was all right.

Flee or fight? She's small. I'm pretty sure I can take her if I choose to fight. But she could have a hypodermic needle in her pocket. I'll lose. Fleeing might be a better idea.

"The results of your breast biopsy came back positive for cancer. The type of cancer you have is called Invasive Ductal Carcinoma Stage I. You are fortunate in that . . . the next step is to schedule . . . MRI . . . surgery . . . this is very early . . . lumpect . . . fortun . . . most women . . . young . . . strong . . ."

The doc's voice kept cutting in and out. My mannequin-face started to melt. She finally stopped talking when she realized I was sobbing.

"I'm going to need to call my husband. He's at work. This is too much information. Can you wait until he gets here?"

"Of course." (Head tilted, eyebrows raised.) "Take as much time as you need. I'll come back and we can continue when he arrives."

Damn. I should have tackled her when I had the chance.

I called my husband and he answered his phone on the first ring. *Did he already know?*

"It's cancer. I have cancer. Can you come?"

"I'll be there in two minutes."

My Knight in Shining Armor mounted his trusty steed, Toyota Sequoia, and as promised, two minutes later, Ludwig was in the room, embracing me.

How did he do that? Desk to parking lot. Steed to hospital. Parking lot to me. That should have taken at least 15 minutes. At least.

"You'll get through this, Terri. We'll get through this. We will."

I felt so safe in his arms.

The young woman doctor returned to the room, along with an oncology nurse named Joan who introduced herself as my "care coordinator." Joan said nothing of also being an Earth-bound Angel, but that's what she became to me. Her gentle and authoritative demeanor put me at ease immediately. She did not tilt her head or raise her eyebrows when she referred to my tumor. Joan looked to be closer to my age, and she spoke to me as an equal, with the respect that her 25 years of nursing experience told her I needed in order to comprehend and embrace my new health status.

A Knight in Shining Armor and an Earth-bound Angel. Sure, cancer bites, but even though I lost the coin toss and got last dibs on picking my team, I saw hope when I looked into their eyes. We were small, but we were scrappy. Team Cancer was not going to take home the trophy. Not this time.

Joan continued to explain the details of my cancer, always cautious to not get ahead of herself. *Now this is a professional.* Even so, my eyes grew wider and my heart raced at the thought of more tests, more anxiety while waiting for test results, surgery, recovery. Radiation. Drugs. More time lost at work. It didn't sound as though my cancer was going to kill me. More likely, fear and anxiety would be the culprits behind my undoing. Panic and tears overpowered me once again.

"Cancer? Who has time for cancer? I get only two weeks of vacation. I can't do cancer. I can't even *afford* cancer! Sick people get cancer. I'm not sick. How am I going to fit cancer into my life?"

Joan took both of my trembling hands into hers. "This cancer is *not* your life. It's a bump in the road. You will find a route around this bump. And I'll help you."

She left Ludwig and me alone for a few minutes, and when she returned she presented me with a beautiful quilted tote bag. Inside the bag was a three-ring binder, neatly organized with tabbed dividers and plenty of clear pockets full of more glossy brochures describing treatment plans, surgery and recovery, breast reconstruction, wigs, hats, and scarves. Last, a beautifully crafted, stuffed fabric teddy bear peeked out the top of the bag. Joan explained that hospital volunteers create and hand sew the bags and bears for the Breast Care Center.

"We've found that some women really enjoy the bears. They bring a sense of comfort and consolation. Just as there are no two cancers that are alike, the teddy bears are each unique, as well. This one's for you."

My jaw nearly hit the ground when she handed me that bag with the bear sticking out of the top. That bear was supposed to *console* me! I obediently accepted it, but I couldn't help but think of it as just that . . . a *consolation* prize. More like a "booby prize."

In my head I was imagining a game show host awarding a parting gift to the loser. *"Here, Terri. You didn't win first prize. After all, you do have cancer. But don't despair. We have a consolation prize for you. A HAND-MADE TOTE BAG AND TEDDY BEAR!"*

Aren't I the lucky one. Here I thought I was going home empty-handed.

When Ludwig and I finally left the hospital, I felt like all eyes were focused on me carrying that damned tote bag. *"Look there. That woman. She must have breast cancer. She's carrying the bag and the bear."* I felt like Hester Prynne from *The Scarlet Letter*, only instead of a red letter A emblazed across my chest, I wore the letters BC (in pink, of course) for breast cancer. That bear would bring me no comfort. No offense intended, but that tote bag and bear would never find a place in my heart, or my house for that matter. I planned to return both on my next visit to the hospital.

Ludwig walked me to my car. "I'll see you at home. Are you okay to drive?"

"I just remembered. I have to go back to the office. I told Helen I'd be back within the hour—it's been almost two-and-a-half. She probably suspects something by now."

"Can't you call her from home?"

"I should tell her in person. She's not just my boss, we're friends. I won't stay long."

"Promise?"

"Promise."

Chapter 3

Marie was at the reception desk, covering the switchboard for me while I was gone. I was exhausted and not up for sharing my news with anyone other than Helen. That's what office grapevines are for.

"Hey, Marie. Thanks for covering phones. I didn't think I'd be gone so long."

"No problem. Helen's in her office."

How does she know I want to talk to Helen?

"Thanks. That's where I'm headed."

Helen popped up out of her chair when she saw me approaching her office.

"Come in, Terri. Have a seat." The pitch of her voice was a few octaves higher than usual. "Let me get the door."

Even with the door shut, we were still visible because two of the walls that enclose her office are glass. It was late in the day, and most of my co-workers had already gone home, but a handful of curious onlookers glanced nonchalantly our way. Suddenly everyone had the urgent need to stroll by her office to replenish paperclips from the supply room or throw a snippet of paper into the recycle bin. It was unusual for Helen's door to be closed; that was the first red flag that something was up. Marie manning the switchboard so late in the day was the second red flag. With an office population of 30, everyone knows everyone's business—everything from lumps in your Thanksgiving gravy to a lump in your breast—it all becomes public knowledge eventually.

Helen and I sat across from one another in silence. She waited politely for me to talk, absently moving items around on her desktop, smoothing her blond hair, lacing and unlacing her fingers. I had rehearsed in the car how I was going to tell her, but now the words were lodged in my throat. I took a deep breath and smiled. Not an "I-just-won-the-lottery" smile; more an "I'm-in-deep-doo-doo" smile. The kind kids use when they spill their grape juice on the living room carpet.

Always the optimist, Helen burst out, "Oh, thank God. Everything's good then?"

Damn. She misread the smile.

"Not quite," I answered. My face turned red as I pushed against the strength of my panic.

"Tell me."

"My results came back positive. It's cancer. Stage I."

"Stage I?"

"They tell me it's treatable and beatable."

"That's good then. You caught it early."

"It's still cancer." I couldn't hold back the tears. "I have breast cancer."

She swung around the desk, and as she sat in the guest-chair next to me, we clumsily embraced in a hug, both of us crying.

Helen broke the hug first, and she held my shaking hands. "I have to pray. Let's pray. 'Heavenly Father, please take Terri in your loving arms and protect her from fear. I know you can't take away her cancer, but please release her from her anxiety and surround her with your love. She's a woman of faith, just like me, but now more than ever, she needs to feel your presence.'"

How does she do that? The words just spill out of her. I wish I could pray like that.

I went into more detail about my prognosis and treatment plan, but I kept it brief. Besides, I didn't really know much anyway. We shared a few more tears, hugs, and nervous smiles.

"Go home. Marie will close the switchboard. Don't worry about us here."

"Thanks, Helen. I'm going to take you up on that offer. I'm so tired from all this crying. I just want to close my eyes and pretend the last three hours never happened."

"I didn't even ask. Was Ludwig there with you?"

"Not at first. When the hospital called this morning and told me they had to see me in person to share my test results, even though my gut was telling me to call him, I was hoping for good news, so I didn't. If the news was bad, I thought I'd be able to handle it on my own."

"So does he know?"

"I started to melt down a few minutes into the doctor explaining my diagnosis, so I called Ludwig at work and he jumped ship and rushed over. He knows as much as I know."

"You're so lucky to have a husband like him."

"No kidding. I thank God every day for bringing him into my life."

Helen and I stood and shared one more hug. A few more stragglers walked by her window as they left for the day, tilting their heads and raising their eyebrows, silently telling me, "so sorry." The grapevine was in full bloom.

On the way home, I kept rolling Joan's words around in my head. Bump in the road. Find a way around it. As well-intentioned as she was in using that analogy, it just didn't fit. My cancer wasn't a bump in the road. A bump can be maneuvered around or over, or kicked out of the way. My cancer was not a bump. It was a lump. A lump in my road. The kind of lump that had to be obliterated. Blasted. Completely annihilated. From what I knew, cancer was a cheating, stubborn opponent. I would need my Earth-bound Angel, my Knight, a kick-ass road crew, and a load of prayers, faith, TNT, and TLC.

By the time I got home Ludwig had already started supper. "I thought you weren't going to stay long."

"Was that long?"

"Longer than I thought you'd be. How'd it go?"

"Not easy. Lots of questions, tears, hugs. She prayed. I listened."

"Did you have to go into it with anyone else in the office?"

"No, thank God. A handful of rubberneckers saw us crying in her office. Most everyone knows I had the biopsy and was waiting for the results, so they've probably put it together by now."

"That's so rude," Ludwig said. "They couldn't respect your privacy?"

"Normally, I'd agree. But honestly, I don't think they were nosing in to be rude. I read it more as concern."

"Whatever. Supper's almost ready. Go change into your comfies. We'll eat in front of the TV."

I know I already thanked you once today, but thanks again, God, for Ludwig.

Chapter 4

Leftovers always taste better when someone else heats them up for you. Neither of us spoke while we ate, a "Friends" rerun the only sound in the room. We both stared blankly and chewed through the drone of canned laughter and endless stream of commercials.

I was the first to break the spell. "Okay, Ludwig, so now we know. It's cancer. When do we tell the kids? They know I had the biopsy. They'll be waiting for me to call with the results."

"We should call them tonight. We'll set up a three-way conference call and tell them both at once."

Ellie was in her junior year at UW Madison, and Karl in his freshman year at UW Eau Claire. They were both in such positive places in their lives, and the last thing I wanted was for my cancer to sideline them. In their 21 and 19 years, they had never known us to be anything but healthy and physically fit. They'd never seen Ludwig or me vulnerable to anything as serious as cancer . . . we barely got colds!

"They're going to freak. I don't know how I'm going to get the words out. They're both right in the middle of studying for exams. I don't want them to panic. Maybe we should wait until we know more about my treatment plan."

"No, Terri, I don't think so. We know enough to get them on board with us. Exams or not, they need to know. Now."

"They'll be scared. It's not enough that they think *they're* immortal. They have us in that category, too. We've always been there for them. How could they even come close to imagining their lives without both of us being only a breath or phone call away?"

Ludwig agreed. "Yeah. Our parenting definitely earned us an 'A' for attentiveness."

"We appointed ourselves their rocks. Unfortunately, I'm not sure we showed them that even rocks erode. Maybe we were as delusional as they were and actually thought we'd never get old or tired or sick. Did we screw up?"

"Number One. No, we didn't screw up. Being their rocks gave them stability. They are who they are today because we gave them stability. It doesn't mean we did the work for them. They were the ones swinging the bats and running the bases. And they had us to lean on when they struck out or climb up on when they hit a homer. That's what rocks are for."

"Wow, Ludwig. You've been hanging out with me too long. You're starting to get darn right metaphorical! Is there a Number Two?"

"I'll take that as a compliment, and yes, there's a Number Two. There's no crime in parenting with attentiveness. Giving them our attention showed them they mattered. What kid doesn't want to feel like they matter?"

"But with us always focusing on them, did we teach them how to look up and focus on others? On us? Did we teach them how to deal with something as big as, 'Mom has cancer?'"

"I think we did. Yeah, they come across as self-absorbed just like most of their generation, but I'd put money on while we were raising them they were listening. And watching. If anything, they learned through osmosis."

There was no hesitation in Ludwig's voice. Only he could use a word like "osmosis" and not sound like a scientist. His confidence blanketed me with calmness.

Chapter 5

No matter how many times I rehearsed the words, *"Hi kids. My biopsy came back positive for cancer,"* I could not finish the sentence without breaking down into tears. I didn't want them to be afraid. I wished I could tell them in person and look into their eyes; Ellie's soft, chocolate brown, and Karl's blue-green, just like mine. Looking into their eyes would lead me directly to their souls. I would know their true reaction.

"Hello?"

"Hi, Ellie. It's Mom. Wait a minute, honey. Dad'll get the other phone. And I want to hook up Karl so all four of us can be on at the same time."

"Wow, Mom. You know how to set up a three-way conference call?"

"I beg your pardon! Yes, your mom is turning into a real techie. Last week I even figured out how to turn on the TV!"

"Hi, Karl. It's Mom."

"And Dad."

"And Ellie."

"We're on a three-way conference call? When did you learn how to do that, Mom?"

"You kids must think I've been asleep for the last twenty years. I know how to do a lot of things."

"Do you know how to turn on the TV?"

"OMG! Yes, I know how to turn on the TV. "

"Ellie, she said OMG. She's talking in text-language."

"Okay, are you two done making fun of your mother? Ludwig, would you please control your children?"

"Oh, so now they're *my* children."

"What's up, Mom? Why are we all on at the same time? Did you get your results?"

Show time.

My heart was beating in my throat, and my head felt like it was going to explode. Ludwig silently motioned from across the room and whispered, "Tell them."

I took a deep breath and got my mom-legs underneath me before answering my daughter's question. This would be one of those phone calls the kids would remember. The kind they'd play back in their memory. If I panicked, they'd panic. It was up to me to take control and ease the words out calmly, the way air escapes from a tiny hole in a balloon, slowly, gently, *hisssssss.*

"Ah, yeah. I did get the results. Dad and I got home from the hospital a few hours ago."

Another deep breath. Swallow. Pause. Hisssss.

"The biopsy came back positive for cancer. But the good news is that it's Stage I. That means we caught it early, and it's very treatable."

Deep breath. Swallow. Wait for their response. Hisssss.

"What does 'very treatable' mean?" I could hear the "budding scientist" in Ellie's voice.

"Well Ellie, Dad and I don't know a lot of those details yet. I have an oncology nurse assigned to my case, and she told us the kind of cancer I have is usually treated with surgery, then radiation, and in some cases, five years of drug therapy."

"No chemo?"

"Not usually. From what I understand, chemotherapy is used more for cancers that have spread to other parts of the body, and from what we know so far, that's not me. Karl, you still there?"

"Yeah. I'm here."

Like water simmering in a tea kettle, my tears were just seconds away from reaching their boiling point. I squeezed my eyes shut and held my breath trying to will the tears away. I would not let the kids hear me starting to lose control.

Ludwig jumped in. "We don't know a lot right now. This is all new to us, but we're asking a lot of questions and kind of learning as we go. Everyone at the hospital's been really nice and patient."

Ellie asked, "What happens next?"

I shook my head, "no." I still wasn't ready to talk.

"I think they told us we'll need to schedule an MRI scan."

"What does the MRI do?" Finally, Karl's voice.

"An MRI will show if there are any other areas close to the tumor that could also be cancerous."

"Cancer cells actually show up on the scan?"

"No, you can see cells only through a microscope. MRI is kind of the Big Daddy of imaging equipment. A radiologist will read the scan, and if any tissue is highlighted, they usually do a biopsy to test the tissue."

"Do biopsies hurt?"

He sounds concerned. Is Karl turning into a young man?

I managed to breathe myself down to where I could talk again.

"Well, let's just say they're no picnic. I had to literally climb up a little ladder onto an imaging table that's supposed to be comfortable, but doesn't even come close. We've tent-camped on softer surfaces."

"Like that campsite at Crystal Lake that had rocks every six inches and Dad couldn't find a flat place to pitch the tent? Remember?"

"Sure do, Karl. Trust me, the campsite was more comfortable than the biopsy table. After what seemed like endless wiggling into the exact position they needed me to be in, they told me to freeze and lie perfectly still. That's impossible, because the exact minute they told me not to move, I felt a cough coming on."

"I know what you mean. I was always *terrible* at freeze tag."

"Karl, let Mom talk."

"It's okay, Ellie. Finally, the techs and radiologist started talking in hushed tones while sticking me with needles. The whole time I wondered what in the heck they were talking about. Recipes? Investment strategies? Every once in a while they seemed to remember I was on the table, and they came out with a too-loud-as-though-I-was-deaf, 'Terri, you're going to feel a tiny prick. Hold your breath.' Tiny prick? I don't think so! Like I said, it's no picnic."

"I've actually been on a few picnics like that."

My son, the comic. Karl, you always know how to cheer me up.

I started to giggle.

"So Ellie, if anyone ever tells you they have to stick a needle in your boob, make sure they're wearing a white lab coat and have a certificate hanging on their wall, *'cause it hurts like HELL!"*

"You got it, Mom. 'Holster that needle, Lab Rat. Show me your papers!'"

Ludwig just shook his head, while the kids and I laughed and snorted like idiots. I knew that look on his face: *Terri, you got the gift.*

Man, it feels good to laugh.

"Okay, now that we've got that out of our systems, do either of you have any questions or concerns about any of this?

Are those crickets I hear chirping?

"Ellie?"

"You said no chemo, right?"

"As far as we know, that's right, no chemo."

"How about you, Karl. Anything?"

"Not really. When do you think you'll have the MRI done?"

"Probably sometime next week. This whole process has moved along pretty quickly. I think cancer gets you to the head of the line."

Ellie asked, "Are you scared, Mom?"

"I'd be lying if I said I wasn't a little bit scared. It's hard to explain. I guess I've seen enough friends of mine get hit with cancer that I never really thought it couldn't happen to me, too."

"You mean you thought it was inevitable?"

"No, not inevitable. More like *realistically possible*. The truth is, no one gets through life unscathed. The last really big bomb in my life was when your Aunt Paula died, and that was eighteen years ago. Dealing with her death was a huge cross. God helped me carry that one, and I have faith He'll help me carry this one, too."

I was trying like hell to hold back my tears. Playing the role of the ever-fearless Supermom, dodging bullets and leaping over tall buildings wasn't as easy as it used to be when the kids were young and gullible. I played my "God card" knowing full well that was the quickest way to end a conversation or change the subject. Born and raised church-going Catholics, Ellie and Karl proclaimed themselves as "skeptics" three summers ago. *Teenagers. Who needs God, right?*

"Well, I should get going, Mom. I've got some studying to do."

Studying? Karl? Is that you?

"And I was right in the middle of doing laundry when you called me. I'd better rescue my clothes from the washing machine before someone steals 'em."

Laundry? Ellie? This is Mom you're talking to!

"Okay, I understand. We'll talk soon. Please, *please* don't worry. I'm going to be fine. I know cancer sounds scary, but remember, I get to live at the end of all of this. It's a lump in the road, that's all."

"Cool, Mom. Did you just make that up?"

"Thanks, Karl. Yeah, on the way home from the hospital."

"A lump in the road. Better than a sharp stick in the eye, right?"

"Way better."

Laughing again. If anyone's got the gift, it's Karl.

"I love you. Have fun with your studying and your laundry. Ellie, don't forget to separate your whites from your Bucky Badger *REDS!"*

"Very funny. Love you, too, Mom. Love you, Dad."

"Love you too, kids. Drink your water. Make good choices."

That was sure to crack the kids up. Drinking plenty of water was Ludwig's cure for anything and everything. He hardly ever closed a conversation without telling them to make good choices. It was his signature sign-off.

Ludwig and I hung up the phones. And I broke down. Again. A day from hell.

"That actually went better than I thought it would." My husband, the eternal light at the end of every dark tunnel.

"You didn't hear fear in their voices?"

"I wouldn't call it fear. More like concern. How could they not be concerned? You're their mom. I'd be worried if they *didn't* sound concerned. Let's take a break from this."

Music to my ears.

Chapter 6

The MRI scan followed one week later.
Another new experience. More time off work. I was
warned by the radiology technicians that I might feel
claustrophobic once inside the imaging tube, and that
the process was a bit . . . noisy. I would have to lie
perfectly still. *No kidding?* Did I have any questions?

Yeah. Number One: How much is this *test
going to cost. And Number Two: Are you sure this is
necessary?*

Earplugs in place, I lay still as the table slowly
fed me into the MRI tube. The fireworks began. Holy
jackhammer! We can send a man to the moon but can't
muffle the noise from a multi-million-dollar piece of
imaging equipment? Feeling confined was the least of
my concerns. Permanent hearing loss was more like it!
This whole cancer thing was really starting to get on my
nerves.

Two days later I called the hospital for my MRI
results.

"Thank you for calling, Terri. The scan did
show an enhanced area of tissue about four inches in
diameter."

Pop! A bright, white light. Buzzing behind my eyes. Shortness of breath.

"Enhanced area of tissue?"

"There's no reason to panic at this point. MRI is so sensitive. It could be a shadow from your hematoma. That bruise is pretty severe. There could be any number of reasons why this area is enhanced. We'll send the results to your surgeon, and she'll be in touch with you with her recommendation."

No reason to panic at this point. Really. Not at this *point. I feel better already.*

More waiting. More anxiety. More darned shadows.

Toward the beginning of this whole nightmare, I was advised to find a breast surgeon. At a very minimum, a lumpectomy loomed in my future. The Breast Care Center gave me a few recommendations. "Find someone you feel comfortable with. Someone you can communicate with."

You mean someone I would trust cutting into my breast with a sharp instrument?

I had a consultation with a male surgeon, and somewhere between our handshake and our next two sentences, I wanted to attack *him* with a sharp instrument. We were not a match. I decided from that one meeting that I would rule out all male doctors. Call me a sexist. I've been called worse.

Next on the list was a female surgeon. My husband and I met with her, and contrary to my prior consultation with "Dr.-Honestly-You-Women-Make-Such-a-Fuss-About-a-Simple-Lumpectomy-Procedure," we both felt at ease with her. She wasn't what I'd call a girly-girl, but she seemed to have just enough estrogen to at least appear somewhat empathetic. Heck. She had breasts. And from what I could see, she had two of them. I figured if anyone could embrace my situation with even a little compassion, she could. Dr. Gallos's name was added to my team roster. Now we were three: Knight in Shining Armor, Earth-bound Angel, Dr. Gallos. And well, me, of course. A team of four.

True to the radiology technician's word, Dr. Gallos called me at work the next day to further explain the results of the MRI scan.

"As you know, Terri, the MRI showed a rather large, enhanced area of tissue very close to the area that we had originally biopsied."

"So I heard. What does that mean, exactly?"

"Well, it could mean a number of things. You still have that hematoma from your biopsy, and it could be that it's casting a shadow on the surrounding area of tissue. We want to be very sure the tissue in question is not cancerous, because if it is, we would be looking at surgically removing more than a lump."

Sweet Jesus.

"How much more?"

"It would depend. Could be a partial mastectomy, could be the entire breast. Before we even go there, though, we need to do another biopsy. An MRI guided biopsy."

Good God. Another biopsy. In one phone call, I went from removing a lump in my breast to potentially hacking off the whole thing. What is going on? This all started with a shadow almost undetectable to the naked eye. I felt like I was in some kind of Alfred Hitchcock movie. Or in an episode of The Twilight Zone. Anger, frustration, confusion. If this phone call weren't taking place at work, I would have thrown an Academy award-winning temper tantrum.

What in Sam Hell is going on here? Are you messing with me?

"I'm going to give you the number to call to schedule the biopsy. Let's just take it one step at a time, Terri. First the biopsy."

Maybe letting Dr. Gallos sit on the team bench with us wasn't such a great idea after all.

I was beginning to feel like one of those little plastic markers on a game board, obediently moving from space to space:

Spinnnnn. Move forward six spaces: You have Breast Cancer!

Spinnnnn. Take the slide to the Red Zone: Biopsy Time!

Spinnnnn. Another Shadow: You Earned One More Biopsy!

Spinnnnn. Sorry: Lose a turn.

Lose a turn. Lose control. Lose a breast. Lose my mind.

Chapter 7

I obediently scheduled the biopsy. Did I actually think I had any choice in the matter?

Whoever invented the MRI guided biopsy procedure clearly had a dark side. Like the kid we all knew in our neighborhood who got a kick out of pulling the wings off flies. Or frying ants underneath a magnifying glass. Demented. Twitchy. Off. Combine the confinement of an MRI tube, the eardrum-splitting noise from the scanner, two radiology technicians, one radiologist, *sharp needles,* and having to lie perfectly still for what seemed like an eternity, and you pretty much have the procedure in a nutshell.

I was fed in and drawn out of the MRI tube so many times I felt like a carriage return on an old manual typewriter. In for imaging, out for measuring and needle sticking, in for imaging, out for needles. In. Out. In. Out. "Hold perfectly still, Terri. You're doing great. We're almost finished." The noise, the biopsy needle, the hard table, not being able to move even a fraction of an inch. I almost made it to the end without crying, but everyone has their breaking point, including me. Crying without moving is a feat. For that I could be proud.

Note to self: Find the name and address of the inventor of the MRI guided biopsy procedure. Contact same.

I couldn't get off that table fast enough. The effect of the pre-biopsy tranquilizer I was required to take had nearly worn off. As a precaution against another hematoma developing, a nurse bound me up tightly, tucking a tiny ice pack into the Ace bandage.

"Is my husband out there?"

"He left for a little bit to pick up a prescription for your pain medication, but I'm pretty sure he's back. I'll go check while you finish getting dressed. Pull the cord on the wall if you need me."

I found my way to the waiting area, and Ludwig was all set and ready to go.

"Get me out of here, Ludwig."

Spinnnnn. Advance to home.

Chapter 8

I was getting used to the routine. Lose time at work. Endure a procedure involving a hard table and sharp needles. Go home. Wait for a technician or doctor to call with the results of the procedure. No matter how many times I repeated the process, the anxiety that held hands with the waiting never got any easier.

This wait was a heavy one. The results from the MRI biopsy would reveal if there was additional cancerous tissue present. The original strategy to remove a lump could turn into a partial or possibly full mastectomy. Potentially losing a breast was one thing. The challenge of having to kill a larger field of cancer was the real issue. This time the stakes were high. For now, I would make my world no bigger than me stretched out on my big, green sofa, in the quiet security of my house, with Ludwig eight feet away at the dining room table. The gentle, rhythmic tapping of his fingers on his laptop soothed me to sleep. (Or was it the pain medication?)

I was lucky enough to get a call from Dr. Gallos the following morning.

Lucky?

"Good morning, Terri. I have your results. Can you talk?"

Can I talk? No, call me back in three years. YES, I CAN TALK!

"Sure. What did the biopsy show?"

"As it turns out, the enhanced area we biopsied showed no cancer. We drew several samples, and they all tested negative. Just as I suspected, that area was probably highlighted due to your bruise casting a shadow. We're good to go with the lumpectomy. I'll transfer you to Kelly, and she'll set you up with a surgery date."

I couldn't speak. I was in complete meltdown mode. Body shaking. Tears spilling. Heartbeat racing. You'd think I'd just earned a shot at the cover of Sports Illustrated Swim Suit Edition!

"Are you there, Terri?"

"Yes, I'm here. That's incredible news."

"Well, we had to be sure. And now we are. Did you want to schedule your surgery date now, or should I have Kelly call you back?"

"Now is good. Thanks again. This is good, good news."

My surgery date was a full two-and-a-half weeks later. I had a whole laundry list of things I needed to tend to before my cutting day, one of which was to get the thumbs up from my general practitioner that I was healthy enough to undergo surgery.

Hmmm. I have cancer. If after a physical exam we find I'm healthy enough to undergo surgery to get rid of it, then how did I get it to begin with? Ironic.

So much to do, so much to think about. Make a To Do list. Coordinate more lost time at work with my co-workers. Grocery shop. Pay the outstanding bills. Get a haircut. Buy new pajamas. Write love letters to the kids and Ludwig in case I die on the table. Whip up a list of my jewelry outlining who gets what. Leave good notes for Ludwig on what the hieroglyphics and color codes in the checkbook register mean. Stop dieting. Eat sugar. Do the laundry. Leave the ironing *(good "grief-therapy" for Ludwig)*.

As far-fetched as it was to think a simple lumpectomy surgery could kill me, I found myself preparing for that tiny "what if."

"Terri, slow down. You'll make yourself sick from worry. You're not going to die. Dr. Gallos has done hundreds and hundreds of these procedures."

"Stranger things have happened. People die all the time from simple surgeries."

"What people? You watch too much TV."

"Anesthesiologists screw up all the time. What if I get one that got only C's on his or her report card?"

"What does 'all the time' mean? Where are you getting your facts from?"

I didn't have an answer. There were no facts. Just fear. Tears welled up in my eyes.

"You're not going to die. You've got way too many church-ladies praying their rosaries for you. I saw your To Do list. New pajamas and a haircut is one thing. Explaining the secret language in the checkbook register to me? Forget it. I don't want to know. You're not going to die."

Either way, I'm not doing the ironing.

Chapter 9

Waiting for my surgery date was like watching a toddler trying to tie shoelaces. The day couldn't come soon enough. It wasn't that I relished the idea of having a plum-sized chunk of tissue removed from my already-too-small breast, but completing that step would allow me to take the next step in my treatment. I had come to accept that I was on a road with a proverbial lump on it, and now I wanted nothing more than to rev my engine and bump that sorry lump to the curb. Anyone who knows me knows that I'm a sore loser, and defeating cancer was not a game I had any intention of losing.

On the Sunday before my surgery date a parish friend approached me before Mass began. I had confided in Dee about my cancer when I was first diagnosed in January, and had been keeping her up to date on my progress. From our past conversations, Dee knew that I was nervous about the surgery. She also knew that I was a woman of faith, since I had companioned and served dozens of parish members over the years through our church's bereavement ministry.

"How are you doing, Terri? Your surgery date is coming up this week, right?"

"It is. Thursday morning. I'm so afraid, Dee. I can't breathe."

"What are you afraid of?"

"I'm afraid I won't wake up. That I'll never see my kids and Ludwig again. That something totally bizarre is going to happen and kill me while I'm on the table."

I started to cry. Dee hugged me.

"Terri, you should have Father Art anoint you after Mass."

"Anoint me? Isn't Anointing of the Sick for people who are dying?"

"Heavens, no. That's Last Rites. Anointing of the Sick is the ceremony for people who are on their way to *recovery*."

"I don't know, Dee. I've never really felt a connection with Father Art. I'm not sure I would gain any comfort from his anointing me."

"Father Art is only part of the ceremony. Parish members also gather in prayer. I've been part of many of these blessing ceremonies, Terri. It's a powerful experience. I really think you should give it a try. You've got nothing to lose."

Reluctantly I gave her the go-ahead. Dee gave me a big hug and fluttered off to find Father Art before Mass began, to arrange the ceremony.

Church-ladies.

I was preoccupied through most of the Mass, wondering what this anointing was all about. What if I didn't feel the sacramental healing vibes during the ritual? Should I fake it? Would Father Art be able to tell if I was faking? Heck, even if I did put on a good act, God would know I was a fraud. That wouldn't be good. This was no time to tick off God. Not now.

Mass ended, and I invited our church-friends-from-the-second-row (Ludwig and I *always* sat in the first row) to my anointing party. As the church started to empty, Father Art, Dee, Ludwig, and a handful of friends started forming a prayer circle at the back of the church. I sat in a chair in the middle. A few more parishioners surrounded me, some of whom I knew, others I did not. Then a few more. The circle grew. Hands joined. A woven chain of friends, acquaintances, strangers, believers.

Father Art joined me in the center of the circle and began the ceremony in prayer, referring to me as, "our sister Terri." He rubbed aromatic oil into my palms and on my forehead, praying for serenity, strengthened faith, healing. Then he placed both of his hands firmly on my bowed head and prayed in silence. Beginning with Ludwig, each member of the prayer circle came forward one at a time and did the same, laying their hands on my head, praying in silence. I could literally feel the power of their prayer coursing through the warmth of their fingertips into my body, my fears falling into my lap through my tears.

The ceremony ended with me joining the circle, all of us praying the Lord's Prayer. I had never felt so loved, so special and connected with the people of my parish, as I did during that ceremony. I could breathe again.

PART 2

———

Baby Steps

Chapter 10

With my spirit healed, the time had come to heal the flesh. I was no stranger to the inside of an operating room. The body is an amazing machine, but it is just that: a machine. Parts wear down, break, stretch out, and tear. The longer you use them, the more maintenance and repair they require. Yet even with a handful of surgeries to my credit, preparing for my lumpectomy felt different. This wasn't a routine lube and oil change. The goal was to remove something toxic from my body. Something with a deathwish. This was a duel: Surgeon vs. Cancer. Winner take all. The stakes were high, and there was no room for error. Dr. Gallos had to win.

The plan was to take Thursday and Friday off work, rest up over the weekend, and return to the office the following Monday. There were no guarantees, but four days of recuperation seemed reasonable. My sister, Vicki, was planning to come down from her home in Stevens Point and stay as long as I needed her.

Vicki called Wednesday night.

"Hi Ter. How're you doing? You nervous? How's Ludwig? He nervous?"

"Vicki! Stop talking! Yes, I'm nervous. And Ludwig's . . . Ludwig. Whoever knows with Ludwig? What time are you planning to get here tomorrow?"

"What time do you think you'll be home from the hospital?"

"Can't say for sure. Surgery is in the morning. Before the lumpectomy even starts, the surgeon has to remove a sampling of lymph nodes from under my arm to have those tested, too."

"Tested for cancer?"

No. Tested for academic intelligence.

"Yes, tested for cancer. Apparently the lymph nodes are kind of the 'party house' for cancer cells after they multiply a gazillion times in your breast. If they get bored, they head on over to the nodes and try to wreak havoc over there."

"How many nodes are removed?"

"As few as possible. The goal is to start with what's called the sentinel node. That's the first one in line in the network. I'll get injected with a purple dye through some kind of air-gun type contraption during the pre-op procedure."

"What's the dye do? Hey that sounds funny . . . dye do, dye do."

"Yeah, funny. Excuse me? These are my *nodes* you're laughing at!"

"Sorry, little sis. Guess I'm just nervous."

"Me, too. The dye is supposed to locate the sentinel node, because supposedly that's where the cancer dudes will go first. If for some reason the dye doesn't find the sentinel, the surgeon has to take a sampling of the next ones in line, removing as few as possible but enough for a biopsy. Chances are if there's cancer in the sentinel node, there's cancer in the rest, and the whole bunch gets ripped out, just like a bunch of radishes, in a separate surgery."

"A separate surgery? You'd have to be cut open again?"

"I know. Bummer. It'd be nice if pathology could do the node biopsy real-time while I'm already on the table, but apparently that's not the way it's done. More revenue to the hospital and doctors if they have to slice you open twice."

"What if there's *no* cancer in the sentinel node?"

"Then they rule out cancer in the rest and leave them all alone."

"I'd be going crazy if I were you. So many 'if's'."

"Who says I'm not? *Crazier than usual.* Ask Ludwig."

"So back to when do you think you'll be home from the hospital?"

"I don't know. Four o'clock? When can you get here?"

"I was going to work most of the day and head out after that. I'll just let myself in if you're not home. Tell Ludwig to call me on my cell to let me know how things are going."

"Will do."

"I love you."

"Love you, too. Thanks for coming down, Vicki. Bring your Barbies and your records. We'll do hair and makeovers just like when we were kids!"

Sisters are the best.

I took one last look at my To Do list before going to bed Surgery Eve. In the end, most of the items did not get done. Deep down, I guess I was banking on surviving the procedure. It was a heck of a lot easier than completing everything on that damned list.

Chapter 11

Morning came way too soon. My stomach was growling from having to fast the night before, and I wasn't supposed to drink anything either, so I was darned thirsty. I wasn't looking to chug a pitcher of beer; all I wanted was a few measly ounces of water.

Are they afraid I'll spring a leak when they poke me with their needles?

The drive to the hospital was a quiet one. Some of the fears that I thought I had sent packing were creeping back into my head. I wanted so for Ludwig to console me with his usual calm and rational way of thinking, but he was silent, too. He wasn't one to start a conversation, but rather more of a reactionary talker. This was our rhythm: I'd blurt out my words. He'd process the weight, texture, and temperature of my words, then formulate an appropriate (or what he thought was appropriate) response. I'd ramble. He'd abbreviate. I'd rip a gut laughing. He'd smile. Right brain. Left brain. A perfect match.

"Do you have Vicki's phone number?"

"I do."

"She'll want you to call her with updates."

"I know."

"And my office number?"

"Yes."

"They're going to want to know if they should start running an ad for a new receptionist."

I giggled. Ludwig grinned.

"And Larry's?"

"Larry's number and the handful of other friends you asked me to call. I'm all set. I have all the numbers. Honest."

"Remember to call the kids."

"I'll remember. I have their numbers, too."

"Ludwig, am I going to wake up?"

"You're going to wake up."

If you say so.

When we arrived at the hospital, we were greeted by a friendly volunteer who walked us through a maze of hallways to Day Surgery, giving us a mini-tour along the way.

"Oh, the staff here at the hospital is just *soooooper.* They'll take good care of you, Terri. Don't you worry about a thing."

"Me? Worried? Do I look worried?"

Extending her arm in a wide, graceful arc, Tour Lady continued, "And Ludwig, did I pronounce that right? *Lud-wig?* This is our new arboretum where you can wait during your wife's procedure. Help yourself to coffee, cookies, snacks. You'll have Internet access, of course, and cable. Stretch out on the lounge chairs. If there's anything you need that's not already here, you just ask one of our volunteers. Don't be shy."

I saw Ludwig's eyes light up when she said "cookies."

Behind our personal escort's back, I mouthed to Ludwig, "Enjoy your free coffee and cookies, dear." Then I smiled. He'd eat them, but he wouldn't enjoy them.

Ludwig stayed with me through most of the pre-op procedure, keeping me company while I settled into my Day Surgery room. What a process! Nurses comin' and goin'. Paperwork to sign. A sedative. More paperwork. An IV for hydration. An IV to knock me out.

"Do you or your husband have any questions?"

"Verify your name and date of birth, please."

"Can you tell me what you're having done today?"

"Which breast?"

"How are you feeling?"

"Sign here, please."

"You're doing great."

"Name? Date of birth? One more form to sign. Questions?"

The whirlwind of people, paperwork, last minute instructions, and questions was unnerving. I prayed the sedative I swallowed would insulate me in silence.

The last two people I saw before I was carted off to the operating room were Dr. Gallos and the anesthesiologist, whose name I never did catch. They looked goofy in their floppy, mushroom-shaped, surgical caps.

Good God. Willie Wonka's Ooompa-Loompas are going to cut me open!

Dr. Gallos's voice was steady and calm.

Robo-doc.

"How are you doing, Terri?"

"Hey, Dr. Gallos. Thanks for asking, but I'm more concerned how the two of you are doing."

"Oh, we're fine. We're just about ready to get started."

"Did both of you have breakfast this morning?"

"Well, I can't speak for Dr. *(I still didn't catch his name)*, but I did. We're all set."

"Then let's everyone do their job today. Find the cancer. Cut it out. I don't care about scars. Just get it and get it all. And make sure I wake up when you're done."

"That's our plan."

They floated out of my room. I was beginning to feel groggy. Heavy.

"Lugwid. Are you still here?"

"I am. Are you feeling sleepy, Terri?"

"Not sleepy. More like drunk. Why?"

"You called me Lugwid."

"I did not. When is Dr. Gallup coming to see me?"

"Dr. *Gallos* was already here. With the anesthesiologist."

"No way."

"You asked them if they ate breakfast this morning."

"Oh yeah. Now I 'member. Could they tell I was drunk?"

"No. You were still all you when they were here. Rude, as usual."

"Hey, is that any way to talk to . . ."

As I drifted off, I felt Ludwig kiss me on the cheek. At least I hoped it was Ludwig.

Chapter 12

Anesthesia is powerful stuff. I closed my eyes. Hours of my life passed without my participation. I was alive on an operating table, but I have no memory to prove I was there. All five senses shut down at one time. Plus memory. None. A surgeon cut into my flesh with a razor-sharp scalpel. How could I not feel that? I guess there were conversations across my body. Doctor to nurse. Anesthesiologist to doctor. How could I not have heard them? I was there. But not. Creepy.

The good news was that despite my fear of dying on the table, I did not. I woke up, just like Ludwig said I would. But my senses were out of sync with what my brain asked them to do. I could see but couldn't focus. I had a voice but couldn't form words. I could hear, but there was no clear definition of sounds. The only sense that thawed immediately upon my re-entry to cognizance was my ability to feel. I felt pain. Severe pain. As though someone was standing on my right breast with a stiletto heel. Sharp, steady pressure. I could make out a blur of nurses just outside my room's door, but I was still too groggy to form words or muster any volume. I watched my hand rise into the air, hoping to send a signal that I needed help. It worked.

"Terri, you're finally awake! What can I do for you?"

I managed to whisper, "I hurt."

"You heard? What did you hear?"

Good God, woman. Pay attention.

A little louder this time, "I hurt!"

"Oh, you hurt. You're in pain?"

I gave her a thumbs up.

"We'll take care of that right away."

Morphine, please.

"Is it over?"

"Yes. You're in recovery now, Terri."

"Does Ludwig know?"

"Yes. He's on his way here as we speak."

I tried to hold back my tears, but I hurt so bad.

"Will you go get Ludwig for me?"

"He's on his way. Hang in there. I'll be right back with your pain medication."

I fell back to sleep.

Then I felt a kiss on my cheek.

Finally, that nurse is back with the morphine.

"Oh, Ludwig. It's you."

"You were expecting . . .?"

"The nurse. I thought it was the nurse. Did she come back with pain drugs?"

"She did. One shot of morphine into your IV and you fell back to sleep."

"Good stuff, I guess."

"Are you still in pain?"

"Not as much. What time is it?"

"It's late. Almost seven o'clock."

"At night? Why am I here so late?"

"I guess the surgery took longer than expected, then they had trouble managing your pain here, in recovery."

"Yeah. I want my money back. Was Dr. Gallos in to see me?"

"She was, but you were asleep. She said she'd come back. I'm thinking we'll be able to leave after she talks to us one last time."

"For home?"

"For home."

"Did you call everyone?"

"What honey? I can hardly hear you. You're whispering."

"Sorry. My throat's so dry. Did you call everyone?"

"I did. Vicki's waiting at the house. Here, take a sip of water."

"I'm so glad this is over."

"Me, too. I didn't think this would take so long. I was starting to worry."

"I woke up. Just like you said I would."

Ludwig held my hand while we waited for Dr. Gallos.

I've never been in Ludwig's shoes. Never had to be the one waiting, pacing, praying. As fairytale as it sounds, I call him my Knight in Shining Armor because he is. He's the guy who has the chair under you before you hit the ground. He always has a fresh handkerchief ready-in-waiting for unexpected tears. An extra jacket or sweater tucked away in the trunk of the car, a band aide in his wallet, Swiss army knife in his pocket. He does what needs to be done, quietly, with no need of recognition. He fills in the empty spaces, laundry, dishes, meals, whatever needs doing, and always with grace. The day may come when I will be able to rescue him from one of life's random acts of unkindness. I'll know what to do, because Ludwig has shown me.

Chapter 13

"Hi, Terri. It's Dr. Gallos. I caught you sleeping again. How are you feeling?"

"Better. The nice nurse brought me drugs. How'd it go?"

"The lumpectomy went well. No surprises there. The goal was to take as much tissue as necessary to remove all of the cancer, plus just a shade more of a perimeter to leave a clean margin with no cancer. We never want to have to go back in for more."

"When will we know if you cut enough to get a clean margin?"

"In a few days. Pathology needs to do their analysis."

"What about the lymph nodes?"

"The nodes posed a bit of a challenge. The dye didn't locate the sentinel node. That happens sometimes. I removed a total of eight. That should provide enough of a sample for pathology to test. If all eight come back clean, then you're set. We'll know that your cancer didn't spread to the lymph nodes."

"Eight. Is that a lot?"

"No. There's dozens more where they came from. You'll have a little stiffness in your right arm, but we'll give you exercises to do while you recover."

"So everything went okay?"

"It did."

"Can we leave?"

"That depends on how you're feeling pain-wise. It's almost eight o'clock. If you need to stay, we'll have to move you out of day surgery and admit you into a permanent room."

Ka-ching. More money.

"Nope. I think I just got better. Better by the minute. We'll leave."

"Good then. We'll send you home with some pain meds and post-op care instructions. A nurse will be in shortly to help you get dressed and sign you out."

"Thanks, Dr. Gallos."

"You're welcome. I'll call you tomorrow to see how you're doing. Go home. Get a little food down, if you can. Take it easy. Ludwig, you're in charge."

He pulled out his crisp, white hanky, and with a quick one-two-swipe to his nose answered, "No problem. I got this."

Chapter 14

I must have dozed off on the way home. The last thing I remembered was rolling through the hospital in a wheelchair. Three-and-a-half-seconds later, we were pulling into our driveway.

"Why are all the lights on?"

"Vicki's here. Remember? She's staying with us for a few days."

"Oh yeah, I remember. Was I asleep?"

"Sound asleep."

"So I didn't nag you about your driving?"

Ludwig grinned. "Not once."

My coat was barely off and Vicki was already hugging me, crying. With her living in Stevens Point, this was the first time we'd seen each other face-to-face since Christmas. After sharing the news of my diagnosis in January, we had talked many times on the phone, but there was nothing like having her beside me in the warmth of my kitchen. The death of our older sister 18 years ago had left just the two of us. Mom is six years into her Alzheimer's. I had no hope for reciprocal love or support from her. Our father was out of our picture years ago. We weren't sure if he was dead or alive. I have no grandparents, uncles, aunts or cousins; it's just Vicki and me. Our whole family history is held between us—we are the end.

"Don't cry, Vicki. I'm fine. Really."

If it weren't for the throbbing, stabbing pain in what's left of my right breast, I'd actually be feeling pretty good.

"I was getting worried. You're home so late," she said, her voice shaking.

"Ludwig called you, didn't he?"

"Well, yeah, but I was still worried. What took so long?"

"Beats me. Nothing ever goes like you think it will. I didn't think I'd be home so late either. Did you find something to eat? How were the roads?"

"Are you kidding me? I know by now not to count on you ever having food in your fridge. What do you people eat, anyhow?"

"Very funny. Now you sound like the kids."

"The roads weren't too bad, for February. You know me. I'd've driven through anything to be here. Forget all of that. I want to know how my baby sis is doing. I can't believe this. It's just too bizarre. *Breast cancer.*" She started to tear up again.

"It could be worse, Vicki. Remember, I get to live at the end of all of this. Not everyone's so lucky. But right now I'm a little dopey and tired from the heavy-duty pain drugs they blessed me with in the hospital. I think I hear my big green sofa calling my name."

By the time Ludwig was done dragging in all the stuff from the car, Vicki was already playing nursemaid, laying me down on the sofa and tucking me in as though I were five years old. Suddenly, I noticed a beautiful gift bag off in a corner of the room.

"Hey, Vickers. What's in the bag?"

"I thought you'd never ask. It's a gift for you. And me. For us. For the weekend." Her face was alive with excitement.

Gads. I was kidding about bringing her Barbie dolls and makeup!

"That's nice. You bought a gift for yourself."

"And you! Dig in!"

Tired as I was, how could I resist diving into that beautiful rainbow of tissue paper?

"Oh my gosh! Robes! Matching pink and white polka-dot robes. They're so soft!"

"Keep digging. There's more."

"Slippers! Pink and white polka-dot slippers. They're so cute!"

"Keep digging. There's more," she said, smiling from ear-to-ear.

"No way. More?"

"Yes, more. Keep digging. The best part's still in the bag!"

I continued foraging through the tissue paper, until I reached something soft at the bottom of the bag.

"A pink and white polka-dot stuffed dog! It's a dog, right?"

"Yes, it's a dog. Isn't he cute? He sort of followed me home."

What a gas. We were giggling like school girls wrapping ourselves up in our new plush robes. Vicki had to help me on with mine, because my right arm was stiff.

"This is the rule: Robe, slippers, and Pink Dog in the room at all times during your recovery. At least while you're on my watch. I happen to know all three have healing powers. Magical, healing powers. Deal?"

"Deal."

Vicki is getting weirder as she gets older. But heck, it's just the two of us. Where would I be without her?

Ludwig busied himself in the kitchen preparing a light supper of soup and toast for me while I settled in. I was still in a lot of pain, but I was also hungry. The soup hit the spot, and within minutes after slurping down the last spoonful, I fell into a deep sleep on the couch.

Chapter 15

Morning light warming my face. Ludwig brushing his teeth in the bathroom. Someone downstairs in the kitchen emptying the dishwasher. Vicki? How did I get into bed? I was on the sofa, now I'm in bed in my pj's. Pain. Pressure. I gotta get out of this straitjacket. I can't breathe. The bandage is so tight.

"You're up. 'Morning. What can I get you? Coffee? Water? Pain pill? How you feeling?"

"Hi, Lud. What time is it?"

"Six-thirty."

"Morning, right?"

"Morning."

"How'd I get up here? I was asleep on the couch."

"Only for an hour or so. Then I woke you up and helped you get ready for bed."

"That's creepy. I don't remember any of that. You didn't sneak any peeks while you were helping me into my pj's, did you?"

"No, no, I was a complete gentleman. How do you feel?"

"I hurt. This Ace bandage and vest-thing-a-ma-jig is so tight I can hardly breathe. Can you help me get out of these mummy rags?"

"Sure. Dr. Gallos said we could re-wrap the Ace a little looser during the day to relieve some of the pressure, but the compression bra has to go back on over it and that's not adjustable. Or negotiable."

"It's all so tight. I think that's why I hurt so bad."

"You hurt so bad because you just had a scoop of tissue taken out of your breast and a bunch of nodes pulled out of your armpit. That's serious stuff, Terri. You're gonna hurt."

Six-thirty in the morning, and I'm already in tears.

"Come on, honey. I'll help you in the bathroom. You'll feel better after you stretch out and clean up a little. Let me run downstairs and get you a cup of coffee. I love you, you know."

"I know. I love you, too."

By the time Ludwig returned with my coffee, I had already unwrapped the Ace bandage. I wasn't able to see what the incisions looked like because of the surgical dressings, but I could see that I was extremely bruised and swollen. Again. The green and purple reminder from my first biopsy in January had barely faded, and now I had another layer of purple on top of that. What a mess.

At least I'm alive.

"I'm going to attempt a shower. If I'm not out in four days, come looking for me, okay?"

"Give me a shout if you need help," said Ludwig.

"Maybe I should wear a whistle around my neck, just for good measure."

What an ordeal. Between trying to keep my surgical dressing dry, and trying to wash my hair with one hand, I regretted ever having started the process. My right arm was so stiff I could hardly lift it over my head.

"Aarrgghhh!"

"What's going on in there?"

"Oh nothing. Just having a good old time," I answered with an obvious tone of sarcasm.

"You need a hand?"

"Two hands. I need *two* hands. I'll be out in a minute."

Think I feel a pity-party coming on.

Frustrated and grumpy, I finished the damned shower and managed to towel myself dry and comb through my tangled rat's nest of hair, still half-coated with shampoo and conditioner. Ludwig waited patiently in the bedroom, knowing that whatever he said to try and comfort me would be the wrong thing. Sometimes silence was the best choice; this was one of those times.

"Well, that was a trip," I grumbled.

Ludwig hugged me, taking a chance with a few words of consolation.

"Hang in there. Tomorrow will be easier. And now to add pain to injury, we gotta wrap you up again."

"Just not so tight, okay?"

"Deal. When we're done here I have to go to the office for a few hours. You and Vicki probably want to get to your 'seesta-seesta' stuff anyway."

I primed a little bit more, talked myself out of the pity-party, then got into my convalescence uniform of pink robe and matching slippers. Onward.

Vicki was already up and clanking around in the kitchen preparing breakfast for us.

"Morning, Ter. Nice robe!"

"My sister bought it for me. And I see you have one, too!"

"I do. Your sister must have incredibly good taste," Vicki chuckled.

"Where's Pink Dog?"

"He's already got his place in front of the TV. I thought we'd start our day with the *Today* show. I've got the sofa all made up for you. Go take your place, little sis. Breakfast is almost ready."

"You don't have to ask me twice."

Vicki and I spent the rest of the day lounging in the family room, alternating between cheesy day-time TV and movies. What a blast. The pain meds added an interesting element to the day, as I drifted from one nap to the next, floating on my inflated rubber sofa, down one long and lazy river.

Chapter 16

As she promised, Dr. Gallos called to check up on me. I didn't have much to report. I wasn't ready to do cartwheels, but the pain was starting to subside. The burning question in my mind was the status of the lymph nodes she removed. Cancer or no cancer? Even though I knew it was too early for her to have heard back from pathology, I took a chance and asked her.

"So, did pathology get back to you yet on the lymph nodes?"

Dr. Gallos responded in her smooth, robo-doc voice, "No, Terri. It's still too soon. We won't have an answer until next week. I'm guessing we'll know by Monday."

"Monday?"

"I know it's frustrating to have to wait that long, Terri. Try to relax these next few days while you're home from work, and get plenty of rest. How did you sleep last night?"

"Not too good. I couldn't seem to find a comfortable position. I tossed and turned a lot. The compression bra is so tight."

"Unfortunately, it has to be. It's important to sleep with it on every night. Wearing it will help reduce the swelling and will hold everything in place so you don't put any strain on your incisions while they're healing. Tuck those tiny ice packs in behind the Ace bandage. That'll help relieve some of the pain and swelling, too. Don't be afraid to take a couple of pain pills before bedtime. They should knock you out. How's your appetite?"

"No problem there. My sis is staying with me for a few days. I've got my silver bell all ready for when I need my next feeding." Vicki overheard me. She shook her head back and forth, mouthing, "I don't think so."

"Well, it sounds like you've got plenty of help behind the scenes. Call my office if you have any questions or problems over the next few days. I'll be in touch with you next week with the pathology results. Keep your spirits up. You're young and healthy, and we caught your cancer early. These are all positives. You'll bounce back. Take your vitamins!"

Was that a surgeon's attempt at humor? "Take your vitamins!" Right. I always took my vitamins. Lot of good they did me. I still got cancer.

"Thanks, Dr. Gallos, I will. Talk to you next week."

The next three days went by quickly. Vicki and I spent hours yakking about our kids and what was new in their young lives. My niece and nephew, Molly and Max, are close in age to Ellie and Karl, but as the four of them grew older, miles, school, jobs, and varied interests began to separate them. Vicki and I constantly impress upon them the importance of staying more connected to one another, especially given the fact that our family is so small. In times of adversity, it's nice to be able to play your "family card" and know someone will be there to hold your hand.

I skipped going to church on Sunday. Showering and primping was still a challenge. I figured God would understand if I prayed from home. In reality, He was probably tired of hearing my voice anyway. I'd turned into a bit of an ornery complainer of late, blaming God and anyone else in my path for my discomfort, my lump, my hairy legs, my stiff arm, my bruised boob, wah, wah, waaaah. Monday was fast approaching, and I'd have to get my act together by then. Behaving like a whiney cry-baby was somewhat acceptable around family members. Co-workers, and basically the rest of the world, would be less tolerant.

As fun as it was lazing around the house, part of me was looking forward to going back to work and returning to my old routine. My position as Director of First Impressions, a.k.a. receptionist, at an independent insurance agency in Hartland, isn't terribly taxing, in mind or body. I also wear the hat of mail clerk and carrier, which means two trips by car each day to the U.S. Post Office, also in Hartland; once in the morning to pick up, and again at the end of the day to drop off. The mail bins could be cumbersome at times, but I knew there would be plenty of fellas in the office to lend a hand if I needed help. The more likely scenario would be that I would simply do it myself. Any woman who's had a couple of babies knows how to tote multiple bundles with one hand (and hip and any other body part that's available) while the other hand is busy doing something else. My right side was still fairly stiff, but functional. I'd manage.

I was also looking forward to getting back to my workouts at the fitness center. My four- to five-times-a-week exercise regimen had taken a beating over the last couple of months for a variety of reasons, starting with two back-to-back biopsies, through my lethargic attitude, and ending with the lumpectomy. I knew I'd be starting all over again building up my cardio endurance and strength training. *That stinks.* The fact remained, I was starting to gain weight, and if I didn't get my sorry butt back on the spinning cycle soon, I'd have one more reason to sing the blues.

My four days of down-time also gave me plenty of time to reflect. A day (an hour?) didn't go by that I didn't struggle with why in the heck I got hit with cancer. Not from a dramatic, beating of the chest, "woe is me" standpoint, but from a fact-based perspective. No family history of breast cancer, good diet, consistent exercise, not a smoker, and only an occasional beer or glass of wine. Hardly ever sick with colds or flu. So why me? How did I get stuck in the cancer line? I learned that we all have cancer cells in our bodies. They usually remain dormant. Unless they don't. What caused mine to turn rogue?

Every medical professional that I'd come in contact with since my diagnosis seemed to be head-over-heels excited about the marvelous advancements made over the years in the detection and treatment of breast cancer.

Sharper technology in imaging equipment. *Yippee.*

Less intrusive surgery techniques to remove cancerous lumps. *Big whoop.*

Better chemo. Safer radiation. More effective drug therapy.

Big. Flippin'. Deal.

I'd be more impressed if someone would get excited about figuring out why more and more women are getting cancer in the first place! Like an uninvited guest, cancer is ringing too many doorbells and invading too many lives. Is the demon lurking in our air, water, or soil? Is it hiding in red meat? Artificial sweeteners? Deodorant? Dry-cleaned suits? What's aggravating our cells into this toxic behavior called cancer? The day I hear a medical professional get jazzed about curing the cause instead of curing the cancer, I'll sing from the rooftops and spin pirouettes in nothing but my undies! Until then, I'll be grateful for all of those so-called advancements—I suppose they're the reason I'm still alive—but I'm not handing out any gold stars. Net yet.

Chapter 17

Vicki and I said our goodbyes on Sunday afternoon. Although she'd never admit it, I knew she had plenty to do before her work week started on Monday. If I had asked her to stay with me another week, she would have dropped everything and stayed, no questions asked. That was Vicki.

"Thanks for coming down, Vicki. You're such an amazing sister."

"I know, I know," she laughed, twisting around, trying to pat herself on the back.

"Seriously. This whole cancer thing would be an even bigger drag if I didn't have you to lean on." I started to tear-up.

"Now don't cry, baby sis. You'll get me blubbering, too."

"I'm still glad it was me and not you."

"What do you mean by that?" Vicki asked, confused.

"The cancer. I'm glad I'm the one-in-eight, and not you."

"Don't be silly."

"I've got Ludwig. You're alone. Everything's easier when you've got a partner."

"Partner or no partner, cancer stinks, and neither of us should have it. Besides, I'm probably the one that's going to get 'The Alzheimer's' like Mumma."

"Do you ever wonder what the dynamic would be if Paula were still alive? Where she'd be in all of this?"

"It's crossed my mind. We'd be back to three-strong instead of two. Paula was always our protector. She would have grabbed that lady doctor that told you your biopsy was positive and slapped her upside her tilted, blonde head!"

Now we were both laughing *and* crying.

"Paula was always so dramatic," Vicki added, blotting her tears with the edge of her sleeve.

"And she exaggerated. Remember how she'd exaggerate the simplest facts? It was the writer in her. Embellished facts were fodder for a story. Everything was bigger than life in her head."

Vicki agreed. "It was easier to act like things weren't a big deal, just to keep her from getting all whipped into a froth."

"She meant well. You can't deny that."

"My guess is that she's looking down on you from that place called Heaven. She knows you have cancer, and she's probably flaming mad that her little sister is going through it without her. She'd want to help." Vicki sounded so sure.

"I know."

It's okay, Paula. Don't be mad. I'm angry enough for both of us. Vicki's doing a great job taking care of me. Ludwig, too.

"Thanks again for sharing all this time with me, Vicki. And for the magical, healing robe and slippers.

You should probably get going before the roads get bad."

One last hug, more tears, and she was on her way, shouting from the driveway, "Call me if you want me to come down again next weekend. We didn't get a chance to play with our Barbies!"

"I'll call if I need you. Drive safe. Love you!"

"Love you, too."

Tail lights.

I promise I'll help you if you get "The Alzheimer's".

Chapter 18

Back to work. Mondays are a drag when you're in good health, even worse when you're not. Lots of delicate hugs and saccharin "that-a-girls" from my co-workers. Bless them all for trying to provide a warm welcome, but I could sense some were uncomfortable, not knowing what to say, how firmly to embrace me, or where to focus their eyes when they spoke to me. Breast-ogling in the workplace was abolished years ago. Why did it seem as though the men were even more conscious of looking over my head (way over) when they spoke to me now?

Maybe I was imagining it.

Come on, guys. Why are you all so nervous? I had a lump removed. I'm still all me. Mostly.

My immediate boss, Helen, started in with what I would and simply would not be allowed to do.

"I'll make the post office runs this week. You are not going to heft those mail bins in and out of your car in this sloppy weather!" she said emphatically.

"Helen, it's not a big deal. I'm just a little sore on my right side. I'll use my left. I'll be fine, really."

"You just take it easy there, Little Missy. At least this week. And if you need to take breaks during the day, let me know. Marie, Chris or I will cover the switchboard for you."

Helen is my closest friend at the office. She and her husband founded the agency 34 years ago, and her son is the president. When I interviewed for the receptionist position three years ago, she and I had an instant connection. We're close in age to one another and both devoted and grounded in our faith. I gained not only full time employment, but also the added benefit of a dear friend. She's a blessing in my life, and she also sits on my bench as a faith-filled member of my team of soldiers, helping me battle through my cancer.

It's good to have a mix of medical and non-medical players on my team. As detached and impersonal as the doctors can be, I need them. Where would I be without their brains? The non-medicals, on the other hand, provide the warm fuzzies. I need them, too. Where would I be without their hearts? My guess is that when I finish my treatment and am liberated from this nightmare, the medicals will drive off in their luxury sedans, and the non-meds will be the ones to stay behind and walk me safely home.

Working a full day proved to be more of a challenge than I thought it would be. The tension of waiting for my surgeon to call with the pathology results weighed heavily. Plus, even in the four short days I was home, I'd grown accustomed to the life of leisure: random naps, sofa-side meal service, crossword puzzles, and blabbing for hours on end with Vicki were the extent of my home-based activities.

Helen asked, "When are you supposed to find out the status of your lymph nodes?"

I kidded her, "Well, that's kind of a personal question, Helen. What's the status of *your* lymph nodes?"

She looked embarrassed. "You know what I mean. Did you find anything out yet?"

"No. My doc thought she'd get the report from pathology today. She said she'd call me as soon as she hears from them."

"The waiting's got to be nerve-wracking."

"Nerve-wracking? That's an understatement. If you or Marie could cover the switchboard after her call comes in, I'd appreciate it."

"Done."

My friend Larry surprised me mid-morning with a visit and a beautiful bouquet of fresh-cut flowers.

Hugs? Flowers? No more trips to the post office? Unscheduled breaks? I could get used to this.

"Oh my gosh, Larry. What a nice surprise! These flowers are amazing."

"Thirty-six years of friendship should count for something. How are you feeling?"

Did I hear his voice shake?

"Other than a little tired, I'm actually feeling better than most of the people around here think I should be feeling. They tiptoe around me like I'm going to break. Honestly, it was just a lumpectomy."

"It's new to them, Terri. Has the company ever had an employee go through cancer treatment before?"

"Not that I know of."

"They care about you. Count it as a blessing," Larry said.

"I do. I know they care. We'll see how long that lasts," I answered, laughing. *"Hey, Terri. Can you*

72

take this eighty-pound package to the post office for me? It doesn't have to go now . . . you can take it on your lunch hour."

"You know that's not going to happen. But speaking of lunch hours, if you don't already have plans, I could come back to the office and take you to lunch. My treat."

"Thanks, Larry, but I think I'll stay in. I'm still waiting for a call from my doctor, and I don't want to get all bundled up and face the elements again. Man, it's cold out there. What did we used to call it?"

"Wicked cold?" Larry recollected.

"That's it. Wicked cold!" I agreed.

I can't believe he drove all the way out here in this crappy weather. Larry hates the cold.

"Consider it a standing invitation. You know you can call on me if you need anything. I know how stubborn you can be, but you don't have to go through this alone. Letting in friends who care about you isn't a sign of weakness. I have plenty of time on my hands now that I'm retired. Call me."

"I will. Thanks again for the flowers and the special trip out here."

Another non-medical on my team. Another friend to walk me safely home.

Chapter 19

The afternoon dragged on. My eyes were glued to the caller-ID display on my telephone in anticipation of hearing from Dr. Gallos.

I'm pretty sure she said she'd call on Monday. It's Monday, right? 262-721-something. I should look up that number. What could take so long? They've had my nodes since Thursday. Get a grip, Terri. She'll call when she knows something.

Finally.

"Is that you, Terri? Dr. Gallos. I didn't realize you were the switchboard operator."

I probably told her that half a dozen times in our short relationship. What is it with doctors and listening to their patients? Are their brains so crammed full of technical data they can't retain simple facts?

"Yes, it's me. What's up? Did you hear anything from pathology?"

"I did. Is now a good time to talk?"

"Give me a second to find someone to cover the switchboard. I'll be right back."

Helen relieved me on the board, and I ducked away into the conference room to resume my conversation with the doc. My heartbeat was racing.

"Hey, Dr. Gallos. I'm back. Thanks for holding."

"I have good news, Terri. Your lymph nodes came back clean."

"Clean as in no cancer clean?"

"That's right. No cancer."

I crumbled into a shaking pile of tears.

"Are you there, Terri?"

"I'm here. I'm just so relieved. Finally, the right answer!"

"Pathology also tested the lump I removed to be sure it had clean margins. Remember, we talked about that?"

"I do. And?"

"There was the tiniest trace of what looked to be a microcalcification on one of the edges of the margin. Our goal was to have completely clean edges."

BAM! Elation to brick wall in four seconds flat.

"So what does that mean?" I asked, trying to control my panic.

"It's such a tiny trace. And we can't even be sure if the calcification is cancerous or not. Probably not worth going back in and cutting a new margin of breast tissue."

"But it could be cancerous. Should we be leaving it there?"

"That's where radiation comes in to play."

"Comes into play how? Radiation would kill any lingering cancer cells?" I was finding it difficult to keep my temper in check. Robo-doc sounded so nonchalant, like this "trace" was no big deal.

Maybe she's just trying to keep me calm.

"That's right. Radiation therapy uses a special kind of high-energy beam to destroy cancer cells, preventing them from multiplying and potentially forming a new tumor."

"Holy crap. How can anyone be sure the radiation will kill every one of them?"

"The statistics for cancer redeveloping in a field that has been treated by radiation therapy are quite low. When you sit down with a radiation oncologist, they'll explain all the details and answer any questions you have about the therapy."

"Huh. So let me see if I have this right. The lymph nodes are clean, so we know the cancer didn't spread beyond my breast. That's good. And the sort of "iffy" margin on the lump tissue doesn't warrant more surgery—radiation should take care of anything left behind."

"That's pretty much it, Terri."

"Well, you're the expert. Let's get started with the radiation. Sooner than later, right?"

"One step at a time, Terri. I'll need to see you toward the end of this week to check on your incisions and see how your breast is healing. How's your pain level been?"

My pain level was just fine until you told me there might still be cancer cells partying in my breast.

"I'm taking the pain medication only before bedtime. How long do I have to wear the compression bra? This thing's a killer."

"If you have a sports bra, you can wear that instead. Are you still swollen?"

"Ha! Swollen and bruised. I don't think I've ever seen a bruise with so many shades of purple and green. How long will that take to fade?"

"It could take weeks, even months. Breasts are slow healers. The color's not the issue, though. The swelling and coagulated blood that's hardened inside your breast to form that bruise is what needs to be almost completely broken down before you can even think of starting your radiation treatments. While you're healing, the next step should be to meet with one of the radiation oncologists on our staff."

"Whoa. Back up the train. A couple of months? In my head I had it that I'd start radiation right away." The pitch of my voice was on the rise.

"It's not as easy as that, Terri. Radiation is an extremely precise process that requires a completely obstruction-free field. Right now, that bruise is your obstruction. When you meet with a radiation oncologist they will go over all of those details and explain the process to you. Hang in there. I know you're frustrated."

You know I'm frustrated? What gave it away?

"Is there anything I can do to speed up getting rid of the bruise?"

Why do I have to draw this stuff out of you, one fact at a time?

"Applying warm, not hot, compresses sometimes speeds up the process. You should be resting when you're not at work anyway, so when you're reading or watching TV at night, give that a try."

Dr. Gallos continued, "If you don't have any more questions, I'll connect you with Kelly so you can schedule a follow-up appointment with me this week. Call me if you have any questions or concerns within the next few days."

"Thank you, Dr. Gallos. I don't mean to sound ungrateful. Like you said, I'm frustrated. It seems for every step forward, I take two steps back. I just want to get this mess over with and get on with my life."

"I understand completely. Try to stay positive. I'll see you in a few days."

"Will do. Oh, and by the way, nice work on the scars—hairline thin. I can hardly see either of them. How am I supposed to get any sympathy with almost invisible scars like these?" I was trying to be funny.

"We do our best. See you at the end of the week, Terri." I detected the slightest bit of chuckle in the tone of her voice. She got it.

Chapter 20

The rest of the day was fairly uneventful. Helen grabbed the end-of-the-day mail bin from me before I could sneak it downstairs to load it in my car. I debated working out at the fitness center. Going directly home and climbing into my nice, warm cozies was definitely winning out, but I was also curious to know how far I'd fallen behind in my level of fitness. The longer I babied myself and stayed away, the harder it would be to don the spandex and face reality.

I'll decide when I pull out of the parking lot. Wherever my car takes me, that's where I'll go. Right, it's home. Left, it's the gym.

Dang. Left.

Wow, the body is unforgiving. I'd been away for nearly four weeks, and the treadmill I was power-walking on was holding a grudge like a scorned lover, resisting every step, relentlessly trying to prove a point that "this is what you get when you ignore me!" I was in a full sweat after five short minutes, angry at the treadmill, angry at the 20-year-old stick-girl running a five-minute mile to my right, angry at my creaking knees, shortness of breath, and most of all at my damned cancer.

Give me a break. There's no need for retaliation. It's not like I was out partying the last four weeks. I was sick!

I swallowed my pride and reduced the speed and incline on my machine, rounding out a full 30 minutes. The poor waif next to me was obviously born without pores. I surmised she was probably drowning internally from trapped perspiration, as she had yet to break a sweat.

Boohoo.

I didn't even attempt working with the free weights. My ego was only slightly more bruised than my breast. I packed up my bag and high-tailed it out of there, hoping none of the regulars saw me panting and sweating from such a puny workout.

I should have turned right.

Ludwig was home from work ahead of me, and he already had supper bubbling on the stovetop.

"Hi, Terri. Why are you home so late?"

"I turned left."

Ludwig looked confused.

"I made the mistake of going to the gym."

"How'd it go?" Ludwig asked, rhetorically. He already knew the answer. My grumpy demeanor was a dead give-away.

"Terrible."

" Didn't Dr. Gallos tell you to take it easy this week?"

"Easy how?

"Easy as in coming home right after work and saving errands and working out until next week."

"She did suggest that, but she also said if I wanted to ease back into my exercise routine, I could, but to take it slow and listen to my body."

"And did you?"

"Did I what?"

"Did you take it slow?"

"I had no choice. I barely made it through a half hour on the treadmill."

"And I suppose you couldn't resist lifting?"

"Are you kidding? After the treadmill kicked my ass I couldn't get out of there fast enough. I was so embarrassed. Next time I'll wear a disguise."

"It's your first day back. I'm not going to tell you to not try again tomorrow, but be a little patient with yourself. You'll be throwing those dumbbells around and spotting for the hulks in no time."

"Very funny, Ludwig."

"Why don't you go upstairs and take a nice hot shower? Supper's almost ready."

"Smells good. What's cookin'?"

"Monday-Night-Surprise."

"My favorite."

Chapter 21

I met with Dr. Gallos four days later. More time off of work. She was pleased with how the incisions were healing, but she reiterated the bruise would delay starting my radiation.

I asked her, "Is that common? To come out of surgery with such severe bruising?"

"I wouldn't say it's common, but it does happen. Remember, you went into your surgery already black-and-blue from your biopsy in January. Traumatizing the breast a second time with the lumpectomy added another layer of hematoma on top of what you already had."

Lucky me.

"Are you trying the warm compresses?"

"I am. Explain again what that'll do?"

I never felt stupid asking Dr. Gallos questions. She was always patient and treated me with respect, no matter how many times I asked her to explain a process.

"The warm compresses will loosen up the coagulated blood that makes up what we see as a bruise. Yours is severe, so it's going to take a while to shrink."

"What happens to the blood once it 'loosens up'?"

"It absorbs back into your body."

"Can't we just empty it somehow? It feels so hard, like there's a lot of pressure behind the incision. Absorbing sounds so slow." If she couldn't hear the desperation in my voice, she was deaf.

"It is a slow process, I'll agree. Occasionally some of the blood can be aspirated, or drawn out, using a syringe. That's done right here, in the office."

"Well, let's do that, then," I blurted. "Stick me."

"We may be able to do that procedure in a few weeks, Terri, but right now it's still too solid. Continue with the warm compresses, and see me in a few weeks for a status check. Have you met with a radiology oncologist yet? I'd recommend either of the two we have on staff."

"I have their business cards, but I haven't made any calls yet."

"Stay positive, Terri. I'll see you in a couple of weeks."

There it is again. "Stay positive." You try it.

PART 3

———

New Normal

Chapter 22

I scheduled a consultation with a radiology oncologist the following week. His office was at the Regional Cancer Center right at the hospital. It would have been nice to have another female medical specialist on my team, but I'd have to make do with a male this time. One of the advantages in choosing an oncologist who was on staff at the same hospital where I had my surgery was that my medical history travelled along with me through their automated medical records system. From mammogram to lumpectomy, they'd have the whole chronology right at their fingertips.

Ludwig met me in the parking lot at the Cancer Center.

"An oncologist. Did you ever imagine in your wildest dreams we'd be meeting with an oncologist?" Ludwig asked.

"Never. What a person won't do for a few hours off of work," I answered.

Ludwig dabbed a tear off my cheek. "Well, let's get this party started."

The Regional Cancer Center was beautiful and welcoming, a sensory experience, not at all what I expected. Soft lighting, a gentle stream of water trickling down a sculpture, walls and upholstery in muted shades of greens, blues, and pink (always pink!), a coffee cart, and the slightest hint of lavender in the air—an essence often used for its calming effect. Before every procedure I'd undergone, the nurses or techs had always offered a lavender-scented cotton ball for me to sniff to calm any anxiety I might have been experiencing. My standard answer, "No, thank you. Got any valium?" always got them laughing.

Despite the spa-like tranquility of the Center, the patients waiting in the reception area told the real story. Some waited alone, others quietly chatted with a friend or family member. Chemotherapy. Radiation. Consultation. People in various stages of cancer waiting for a serving of their treatment-of-the-day on the other side of the counter. A man in a wheelchair, a young woman wearing a wig. Where were they on their road to recovery? Would they recover? What were they thinking as they spied Ludwig and me across the room? By all appearances we were both healthy and strong. I imagined what their conversation would sound like, if they shared their speculations out loud.

I'll bet it's him.

No, it's her. Breast cancer.

No, it's him. Prostate.

Definitely her. Her confidence is an act. She's scared.

He looks scared, too. I'm sticking with him. Maybe it's colon.

No, it's her. See there. He just reached for her trembling hand. Definitely her. The bulky scarf she's wearing on top of her sweater is the give-away. She's hiding her lopsidedness. It's her.

You might be right. Either way, it's a damned shame.

Ditto.

"Terri? Terri Enghofer?"

A nurse calling my name silenced the conversation within my imagination.

Dr. Gates. A new team member on my roster. In baseball, he'd bat fourth: the clean-up batter. He was dressed impeccably in sport coat, crisp dress shirt, tie, pleated trousers, polished shoes, and the slightest trace of cologne. Not particularly handsome, but classy. I guessed he was in his mid- to late-50s. No lab coat, though. I wondered if this guy was really a doctor. The framed certificates on his walls said he was, but where was his lab coat? Aren't doctors supposed to wear a white coat with their name and abbreviated degrees embroidered over the breast pocket? I was already feeling uncomfortable, and we hadn't even shared introductions.

"So Terri, tell me what's been going on with you."

Are you kidding me? Why wouldn't you already know that? You're drumming your fingers right on top of my medical file! It's all in there. Don't you prepare before meeting your patients?

"Going on with me?" I answered, trying to mask how annoyed I was at hearing him ask such a stupid question. Yes, there is such a thing as a stupid question. The doctor-impersonator sitting in front of me had just asked one.

"Well, as I'm sure you read in my medical file, this all started with a routine mammogram I had taken back in November . . ." and I continued my story using the exact dates on which tests were taken, results given, and treatments performed. Dr. Gates appeared to be engaged, though passively, but I was still aggravated as to why in the heck I was using valuable, expensive consultation time to reiterate facts that were screaming for attention under his fingertips.

I summed it all up with a resounding, "That's my story and I'm sticking to it!"

All three of us chuckled.

"You certainly have a tremendous memory for details, Terri."

"So far my brain's all here. It's my breast that's getting eaten alive."

Ludwig shot me a look that suggested I ease up on the sarcasm.

I raised my eyebrows in response.

Ahh, the silent language of married people.

"You have a sound understanding of your condition, Terri. That makes my job, all of our jobs, easier as we begin the radiation phase of your treatment."

That's my goal. To make your job easier.

"That brings up a question, Dr. Gates."

"Shoot."

"Is the treatment we're following the normal course of action for my kind of cancer? Everything I've read consistently outlines: surgery, radiation, medication. Are there other approaches or strategies I should be considering?"

I sensed a subtle change of expression in the doc's eyes. He stopped drumming his fingers on my file.

Don't get excited. I'm not questioning your intelligence. Although I would like to know why you're not wearing a lab coat. Are you a real doctor?

"The course we're using to treat your cancer is the industry standard. Although no two cancers are exactly alike, they do fall into categories. Treatment strategies are designed based upon research, statistics, and results. The protocol for treating your cancer is, as you said, surgery, radiation, medication. We've had a lot of success over the years with that format."

"Seems pretty cut and dried."

"Nothing about cancer is cut and dried. The way we treat it today isn't the way we treated it even 10 years ago. The survival rate for women diagnosed with breast cancer increases every day due to continued advancements in technology and research. Trust me when I say we've come a long way."

My jaw tensed as I ground a chunk of anger between my back teeth.

Ludwig jumped in before I had a chance to grab the doc by his silk tie and share my thoughts on how we've come a long way. "So, tell us about how radiation works." This time his look said, "Go easy, Terri. We need this guy."

I couldn't resist. "I guess I'm still shooting for the experts to find a cure for the cause instead of a cure for the cancer. How far have we come with that, Dr. Gates?"

Of course that would put you out of a job, wouldn't it?

"Not far enough." *Score!* "We'd all like to see a cure for the cause, as you put it. Now, let me explain the radiation process to you and your husband."

Dr. Gates spent the next 10 minutes explaining the technical side of radiation therapy, in encyclopedic detail. When our eyes started glazing over from being bombarded with too-many-facts-in-too-little-time, he took a breath and asked us if we had any questions.

"Wow. Can you break some of that down into laymen's language?" I asked.

"Where did I lose you?" He sounded confused, as though the non-stop stream of mumbo-jumbo that just spewed out of his mouth was as easy to comprehend as folding a sheet of paper in half.

"Did you say something about having to have a total of thirty-three treatments?"

"I did. Thirty-three treatments is the standard protocol."

"Thirty-three treatments," I repeated to be sure I heard it right. "That'll take forever."

Dr. Gates answered, "Not really. About five-and-a-half weeks."

"What? How do you figure?"

"One treatment every day of the week. Excluding weekends, of course."

"Are you kidding me? I work full time. How am I going to swing scheduling a radiation treatment every day of the week? That's just not feasible."

"Unfortunately, that's the reality. Radiation is most effective when it's administered consistently. We do our best to schedule your appointments at a time of the day that works best for you and your work commitments."

"How long does a typical treatment take? What are we talking, here? Tip to finish."

"Tip to finish, you'd be looking at about fifteen minutes."

"Add in my drive time from the office and back again. I'd be looking at about forty-five minutes a day, Monday through Friday."

"That sounds about right."

I was out of responses.

Dr. Gates continued, outlining the possible side effects. Fatigue. Browning and possible burning of the skin. Peeling. Sensitivity. Itching.

Please, tell me more. This just gets better and better.

I managed to claw my way to the top of the muck pile that this oncologist without a lab coat had just dumped on me, and squeaked out a shaky, "So when do we get started?"

"I thought you'd never ask."

Humor? Give me a break.

Dr. Gates finally opened my file, and after what I considered to be a too-quick scan of its contents answered, "Tell me about this . . . hematoma."

He said the word "hematoma" like he was trying to pass a kidney stone. It's a bruise. It's huge, rock-hard, and a stubborn s.o.b. Tell me you know what a hematoma is.

"Yeah. My infamous bruise. It follows me everywhere. I just haven't been able to shake it loose." I wanted my sarcasm to get under his skin, just a little . . . like a hematoma.

No reaction. Damn, this guy is irritating. It's all explained in the file, doc. Can you read? Seriously? I need to explain this?

"I got the heee-ma-tohhh-ma back in January when I had my original needle biopsy. As I understand it, the radiologist was trying to move the needle from one cluster of microcalcifications to another, and broke a bunch of vessels while doing so. He had to take out the needle and end the procedure prematurely to stop the bleeding."

"That can happen sometimes," Dr. Gates answered.

Really? I continued. "After my lumpectomy in February, I suffered more bruising. I'm sensing some concern on your part?"

"A little. Depending upon the severity of the bruise, we could be delayed in starting the prep work for your radiation treatments."

"Prep work?"

"Mapping. Our goal is to direct the beam of radiation as close as possible to the exact spot of where your tumor was removed. This calls for an extremely precise measuring and marking system, known as mapping, so that every treatment is exactly the same as the treatment before. If we measure your breast while it's still swollen and bruised, the quadrants that we set to aim the dose of radiation won't be accurate as the area starts to heal and shrink."

"Interesting. So we wait?"

"We wait."

No one spoke. The silence, albeit only 15 or 20 seconds long, was maddening. Was I waiting for the doc to speak, or was he waiting for me? Or were we waiting for the bruise to shrink? We couldn't possibly sit in silence in that room for the next two or three weeks.

Ludwig cleared his throat. I jumped. Dr. Gates remained deadpan.

Good God. Is this some kind of a contest: "Can You Hear the Hearts Beat?"

"So, what's next?" I finally blurted. Dr. Gates jumped. *Ha! He's alive.*

"Good question. See the receptionist on your way out and schedule an appointment to see me in about two weeks. As that date approaches, if you don't feel the bruise has made any progress, give us a call and push the appointment out another week or so. In the meantime, call my office if you or your husband have any questions or concerns. We covered a lot of information today."

We stood up to leave. "Thank you, Dr. Gates. I guess we'll be in touch."

Be sure your lab coat is out of the laundry the next time we meet.

Chapter 23

Ludwig and I walked to the parking lot without saying a word to each another. I was in such a foul mood, and between the tense look on Ludwig's face and his uncharacteristically quick pace, I sensed he needed the silence.

Is he angry with me? Angry with the doc? Angry with my cancer? It's way past our lunch hour. Maybe he's just hungry. When can I talk?

I caved. "Do you believe that guy? I was *not* impressed. He didn't even have on a lab coat. He looked like he'd just come back from the theater in his dapper-Dan tweed sport coat and silk tie. And what was up with . . ."

Ludwig cut me off. "Terri. What's up with YOU?"

"Me? What's up with me?"

"Yeah, you. Could you have been any ruder? Your attitude. The tone of your voice. The sarcasm! My God, Terri."

"MY attitude? Give me a break. He was twenty minutes late. He was unprepared. I had to explain everything to him. My whole story. Then when he finally woke up, he spoke to us in doctor-ese instead of normal words. What was the purpose of that? To impress us?"

"Face it, Terri. It's the nature of the beast. Doctors don't come with a bedside-manner. It ticks me off, too. We're just going to have to accept it."

"That's you. Mr. Acceptance."

"Don't knock it. Which one of us has high blood pressure? Hint: Not me!"

That was low. "All I'm asking for is a little respect. He sat there so smug and so impressed with 'how far we've come in the treatment and early detection of breast cancer.' As though it was no big deal that I have two breasts that don't match, like the last two socks out of the dryer."

"He was probably more prepared than we think. Maybe he held back because he wanted to see how much YOU knew about your cancer. We can't make assumptions, and we can't judge his medical expertise over whether or not he wore a lab coat."

"Fine." *Not fine. The doc was still smug. If I don't like him the next time I see him, I'm kicking him off the team. He'll be off the bench and into the ditch before he can tie a double-Windsor.*

Ludwig wrapped me up in a hug before we got into our cars to go back to work. "It'll be okay, Terri. I'm not going to let just anyone zap you with radiation. Not one time, and especially not thirty-three times. So far this guy passes the sniff test with me."

I scrunched my nose. "Ooh, you liked his cologne?" Ludwig rolled his eyes.

Chapter 24

Who knew a bruise could cause such a delay? Unbelievable. I was looking so forward to starting my radiation treatments and coming closer to the day I could finally wake up from this nightmare. I was damn sick of cancer intruding into my life. Sick of coordinating doctor appointments into my work schedule, managing the continuous flow of paperwork, having to explain to friends where I was (or wasn't) in my treatment, doubting the efficiency of my doctors, and wondering, always wondering if I'd end up a survivor or a memory. That was the exhausting part. Trying to keep the constant nagging of doubt at bay. I was so tired of hearing people say those words, "You'll get through this, Terri. I know you will." Those words meant nothing to me. They were trite, and unsubstantiated. The more I heard them, the more I wanted to lock myself into a closet and post a sign: You Know Nothing. Stop Pretending You Do. Go Away.

I shouldn't have been surprised that the radiation therapy couldn't start until the bruise was gone. Dr. Gallos spelled that out in my last appointment. But like a kid who just sailed a baseball through the neighbor's kitchen window, I thought if I could run fast enough and hide behind a row of hedges, everything would be okay. Hiding didn't work then. And it wasn't going to work now.

I spent the next month applying warm compresses to my breast, trying to break up the coagulated blood in my bruise. Although the progress was slow, I did start to see some reduction in the size and firmness. I remembered that Dr. Gallos said that if a bruise became soft enough, sometimes the blood could be aspirated through a syringe, so I scheduled an appointment with her. The thought of her sticking a sharp needle directly into my breast did not excite me, but desperation is a mighty motivator.

"Hey, Dr. Gallos. Let's see you work some magic with sucking this bruise dry."

"Well, that's a tall order, Terri, but I'll see what I can do."

She gave my chart a quick scan. "Wow. It's been six weeks since your surgery. Have you had a consultation with a radiology oncologist yet?"

"I did. About a month ago my husband and I sat down with Dr. Gates."

"Oh, Dr. Gates. We go back a long way. He's good."

I'll have to take your word for it. "We've hit a log jam, though."

"Log jam?" Dr. Gallos asked.

"We can't start my mapping until this darn bruise is almost completely gone."

"Well, let's see what I can do to help that along."

Dr. Gallos left the room for a few minutes. *I'll bet she's on her way to the closet that stores the aspiration syringes, rubber gloves, hip boots, goggles and restraints. She had a weird smile on her face when she said, "Well, let's see what I can do to help that along." Maybe this isn't such a good idea after all.*

"Oh. My. God. You're going to stick that big needle into my breast?"

"I know it looks menacing, but honestly, the procedure goes pretty quick. Try to relax. Sometimes it helps to look away."

"Look away? Would that make the needle get smaller?"

I took her advice and turned my head toward the wall. *You've been through worse, Terri. Deep breath.* She was able to extract only a very small amount of blood. What a waste. Three hours of lost time to make up at work, and another layer of disappointment.

"I was hoping for better results, Dr. Gallos. It felt like the bruise was starting to soften up. I've been applying warm compresses every night. I don't know what else I can do."

"Hang in there, Terri. You've made progress. Keep doing what you're doing. It'll break up eventually. We can try this again in a couple of weeks if you'd like."

"I guess. Thanks for trying."

Now I was angry. I'd had it with this damned bruise running the show. I continued to apply warm compresses every night for the next two weeks. Then one morning Dr. Gallos' words, "It'll break up eventually," became a reality. I was taking a shower and noticed a small puddle of blood pooling at my feet.

Egads, where in the heck is that coming from?
Did I cut myself shaving my legs? Stay calm. Assess.
Now I know how Janet Leigh felt in "Psycho."

I'd sprung a leak! The two-inch incision from my lumpectomy had split open about one-quarter of an inch, and a slow but steady trickle of blood was escaping. After I steadied myself from the initial panic, I shouted out a loud, "Wa-*hoo*!"

Ludwig happened to be brushing his teeth in the bathroom at the same time and asked, "What's going on in there? You alone?"

"The dam finally broke!"

"What dam? Do I need to come in there?"

"My boob! The pressure from my bruise finally punched its way through the incision. I'm bleeding! Wa-*hoo*!"

"Quit with the wa-hoo's! Are you okay, Terri? What should I do?"

"I'm fine, I'm fine. Now that I have an opening, I'm going see if I can massage some of the coagulated blood loose."

"Terri, you should stop. This doesn't sound healthy. What if the incision opens more? Get out of that shower and let me see what's going on."

"I said I was fine. I'm fine."

But I was scared. Ludwig was right. What if the cut opened further? Then I'd really be in a pickle— wet, naked, and bleeding—not a good combo. Still, I had to experiment. Just a little. I kept the water running as a distraction so Ludwig would quit yelling at me to stop. My heart was racing as I massaged the bruise, the blood still only a tiny trickle. Then BAM! I went too far, and the dike really did let loose!

"Oh dear!"

"Terri, stop right now. Get out of that shower!"

"This is so cool, Ludwig. The more I massage, the more the bruise is literally emptying out of the cut. All it needed was an opening."

Ludwig opened the shower door and slammed the water off. He grabbed a towel and pressed it to my breast. "Enough. Let's dry you off and see what's going on here. Man, you're stubborn."

"I'm sorry. But I think I'm on to something."

Gross as it was, I found the solution to stomping out my nemesis. For two solid weeks I repeated the process of warming up my breast, then massaging and squeezing built-up blood out of the incision. From an outsider's perspective I may have been construed as warped, but from my side of the fence I was simply doing whatever it took to get rid of the obstacle that was preventing me from starting my radiation. At Ludwig's urging, I reported my "heat n' squeeze therapy" to Dr. Gallos. She didn't tell me to stop, but she did advise me to keep the incision clean and to be watchful that it didn't open further.

I knew she'd see it my way. Women doctors rock.

Chapter 25

I thought I'd seen everything until the day of my long awaited mapping, a collaborative process involving two radiation technicians and my old pal, Dr. Gates.

"You made it!" Dr. Gates shook my hand and gave me a warm welcome.

"I did. Here in the flesh. Today we map, right?" *Glad to see you found your lab coat. You've no idea how close you came to being traded for a real doctor.*

"That's the plan. Let's take a look."

What got into him? Such enthusiasm! This isn't the bore I had the consult with six weeks ago. It's got to be linked to the white coat, like how Clark Kent doesn't turn into Superman until he puts on his cape.

One of the techs walked me over to the table where the mapping would take place. The room was dark except for bright lights haloing the table. All kinds of equipment hung from the ceiling. I felt like Dr. Frankenstein's monster, fully expecting Igor, the hump-backed lab assistant, to limp out from a dark corner of the room.

I lay down on the table and Dr. Gates turned down the white pillowcase (yes, pillowcase) that draped across my upper body.

"You've made progress. The little that remains of your hematoma isn't going to present any problem at all. You're ready."

Am I?

"Randy and LeeAnn are going to start the measuring and marking process. You look nervous," Dr. Gates said.

"I am. As much as I've looked forward to this day, now that it's here, I'm not going to lie, it's a bit overwhelming." My throat was tight, and I could feel tears planning their escape.

"That's understandable. Try to relax," Dr. Gates answered.

LeeAnn added, "You're in good hands, Terri. Randy and I will explain everything we're going to do before we do it, and please ask questions or let us know if you're uncomfortable in any way."

"You've both done this once or twice before, right?"

"Hundreds of times. Honest."

I exhaled a giant sigh of tension and gave them the thumbs up signal. "Okay, then. Do your stuff."

The pillow my shoulders and head rested upon felt like one of those beanbag chairs from the 1970s. LeeAnn asked me to raise my arms over my head and rest them on the pillow. I squirmed a little, trying to get comfortable, and wondered why I was lying on a hunk of noisy plastic filled with beads. Between the meager pillowcase used to cover my waist-up nakedness and the cheap piece-of-junk pillow I was lying on, I wondered where the thousands of dollars I'd already forked over in medical expenses were being spent.

"What's up with the plastic pillow, right?" Randy read my mind. "After you find a comfortable position, a machine is going to vacuum the air out of the pillow, and it'll shrink, forming a custom-fit mold that you'll lie on during each of your radiation sessions. It's the first step toward ensuring that you'll be lying in the exact same position every single time we treat you."

"Ohhhh. Now I get it. What's next?"

I had to ask. Out came the black permanent marker and tattoo gun. Images of a side of beef came to mind (*Chuck. Rib. Loin. Round. Brisket. Flank.*) as I felt the cool tip of the Sharpie pen draw hash marks on my skin. Although I couldn't see exactly what the two taggers used to choreograph their jet black graffiti, I assumed they were using x-rays. It was an odd sensation, being drawn on. LeeAnn and Randy talked quietly over me and about me, but didn't include me, as though I weren't in the room. What kind of diabolical scheme were they plotting?

Igor, get me out of here.

"How do I keep the pen marks from washing off in the shower?"

LeeAnn answered, "That'll happen, eventually. That's why we'll also apply tiny, permanent tattoos, to mark the field that'll receive the radiation. Dr. Gates will check our penned measurements before we set the tattoos."

"My son's going to have a jealous fit when I tell him his old mom got inked."

"Why's that?" LeeAnn asked.

"He begged me and my husband for permission to get a tattoo. We were dead set against it."

"And did you give in?"

"Of course we did. One week before he left for college, he got stamped. I cried for days when I saw that black mark on his ribcage. The perfect baby boy I created, permanently stained."

"I'm guessing it wasn't a heart with the word Mom scrawled through it?" Randy asked.

"Not even close."

"The suspense is killing us. What did he get?"

"A cat."

"A cat as in 'Hello Kitty'?" LeeAnn asked.

"God, no! A cat as in the Halloween kind. You know, a silhouette with an arched back."

"Why a cat?" Randy asked.

"It's the idea of the nine lives that intrigues him. That nothing is forever. I'm guessing he sees the cat as a symbol of hope."

"Wow. That's kind of deep."

"The words 'nine lives' are written in scroll over the cat's back. He designed it, so he's proud of it. Now that I'm over the shock, I think his 'cat tat', as I call it, is actually pretty cool."

"Well, yours will be tiny dots, almost invisible. LeeAnn, what do you think, are we ready to call in Dr. Gates?"

"I think so," she answered. "Terri, are you cold? Would you like a blanket?"

What I'd really like is a shot of whiskey. Got any of that tucked away under a white pillowcase?
"I'm fine, thanks. Still a little shaky, though. The reality of why I'm here in the first place still blows me

away. If there's any truth to the 'nine lives' theory, I'm hoping I can cash in on one of mine just in case I don't come out the other end of this cancer ordeal."

"We can only imagine what you're going through. Randy and I have seen hundreds of women come through this cancer center. The day of your last treatment we're going to tell you what we tell all of our survivors: 'Get lost. We don't ever want to see you here again!'"

"LeeAnn is right. We have a pretty darned good track record, which means we must be doing something right."

"Thanks for the pep talk. No offense, but I'll look forward to getting the boot."

"Dr. Gates'll be in in a few minutes. Sit tight."

Sit tight. Where would me and my body graffiti go?

Chapter 26

Dr. Gates and his white cape flew into the room a few minutes later to review LeeAnn and Randy's pen markings.

"Everything looks good, Terri. LeeAnn will place your dot-tattoos, and you'll be on your way. Do you have any questions?"

"I do. When do the thirty-three days of radiation start?"

"As soon as we can get you on our calendar. I'd guess Rita can work you in starting this coming Monday."

"Rita?"

"You passed her on your way in. Stop at her desk when you leave and tell her your time preferences. She'll work with your availability as best she can."

"I'm still not sure how I'm going to swing coming out here every day with working full time."

"Rita is a master at scheduling. She may even have an early slot available before you start work, or during your lunch hour," Dr. Gates said, making an attempt to ease my stress.

Perfect. I'll eat my peanut butter and jelly sandwich while I'm lying flat on my back getting nuked.

Of course the techs will have to feed it to me since my arms will be locked in place on my customized plastic pillow.

"Any more questions?" Dr. Gates asked.

"None that come to mind right now."

"If you think of anything, call my office."

LeeAnn returned, wielding her tattoo gun. "This won't take long, Terri. I'll get right to the point. You'll feel a tiny prick with each dot. Quick and painless."

I laughed. "You heard the pun, didn't you?"

"Pun?"

"'I'll get right to the point?' Your tattoo gun? Point on the end of it? Be honest, LeeAnn. You use that joke on everyone."

"Okay. You got me. It's kind of my signature."

"Well, I'm up for quick and painless. How many dots?"

"Six."

"Can I choose the color?"

"I'm afraid not. Basic black is the color of the day, but you'll hardly see them, they're so tiny."

"Okay then, fire up that bad boy. If I like what I see, I'll give your name to my son."

LeeAnn was telling the truth. Six black dots formed a permanent rectangular constellation on my chest and ribcage, about 16" across by 6" down. Nothing to write home about, but an indelible reminder that when I was 53 years old, cancer tried to take me down. And lost.

"Explain the purpose of the dots, again?" I asked LeeAnn.

"Once we get you settled onto the table and into your pillow, we'll line up a series of laser beams to coincide with your dots." LeeAnn pointed to camera-like devices mounted from the ceiling. "Those are where the beams come from."

"So the dots act as coordinates?"

"Exactly like coordinates. We don't want to be aiming doses of radiation into your body willy-nilly, so it's critical that you're lying in the same exact position for each treatment. The objective is to saturate the spot where your tumor was removed, but at the same time avoid hitting vital organs and tissue that surrounds that area."

"That doesn't seem possible," I said. "How does the radiation know what to zap and what to leave alone?"

"It doesn't. That's why we have to tell it by programing our equipment precisely to the right target."

"As far-fetched as that sounds, I guess I'm going to have to trust that you and the doc know what you're doing."

"You just concentrate on staying healthy, Terri. Radiation kills every cell in its path—it can't differentiate between cancerous and healthy ones. When cancerous cells are hit, they aren't able to re-boot themselves, but the healthy ones shake their little heads and get right back on the saddle."

"*Go cells!* The body is a pretty cool machine."

"I agree. The cell rebuilding process takes energy, though, so you may feel tired toward the end of your day. It's important to listen to your body and rest when you feel tired. You need to respect the fact that you may not be able to run at your normal pace. That's the hardest part for most women—taking time to rest."

"Are you serious? You mean I have to ditch my workouts and be waited on, hand and foot, by my husband?" *Hmmm. Where did I put my silver bell?*

"That's a little extreme, but it wouldn't hurt to slow down and call on the 'kindness of strangers' once in a while. This is serious stuff, Terri."

"Like I used to say to my kids, 'I'll think about it.'" *Which means: fat chance.*

"Looks like we're all set. You and Rita need to coordinate a schedule. Your first appointment will be a dry-run. That'll be on the first Monday she has an opening. Everything will take place like a typical radiation treatment, but we won't actually be dosing you. Dr. Gates will do a final check of all the measurements, the laser beam alignments, and the rotation of the device that sends the radiation into your body."

"Rotation? What's that all about?"

"You'll be receiving three doses of radiation from three different angles."

"So that's what this machine hanging over me does?"

"That's it. It'll shoot a dose on a downward angle from the left, then rotate and hover over your body to the right for a second dose, then rotate down to your right side and shoot a third dose on an upward angle."

"And where will you be during all this?"

"The radiation techs will be behind that glass window remotely operating the machine that shoots the radiation. It'll all make more sense once you see it in action."

What do you mean? It makes perfect sense. I'm going to be lying on a table, naked from the waist up, and shot with radiation three times while you guys watch from behind the safety of a wall of glass. I get it.

LeeAnn must have read my mind. "It's perfectly safe, Terri. We protect ourselves from the possibility of exposure to radiation because we administer it day in and day out."

"Again, I'll have to take your word for it."

Rita, the master scheduler, was very pleasant to work with. Most of my appointments landed either before work, or within the first hour of my job, which meant I'd potentially punch in late or leave my post at the switchboard and do an out-and-back to the Regional Cancer Center. The worst case scenario would still be only a 45-minute loss of time in my work day.

"How does the schedule look?" Rita asked.

"Not too bad. In a perfect world I wouldn't have to miss any time at work, but then again, if it was a perfect world I wouldn't have cancer."

"I'll keep my eye out for early morning openings. We can tweak the schedule as we go."

"Do appointments generally run on time? Does seven-forty-five a.m. *mean* seven-forty-five?"

"You bet it does. We schedule patients in fifteen-minute intervals. That doesn't leave much wiggle room. All it takes is one late arrival to potentially collapse the whole house of cards."

No pressure there. One bad hair day or getting stuck behind an old geezer in a Buick doing 12 in a 35 could mean a cancelled session.

I kept staring at my copy of the calendar.

"Questions, Terri?"

"One. Why are Monday sessions longer than Tuesday through Fridays?"

"On Mondays you'll be meeting with Dr. Gates, usually after your treatment."

"*Every* Monday?"

"Every Monday. It gives him a chance to address any concerns or questions you may have as the weeks progress."

You mean it gives him a chance to bill my insurance company once a week for a face-to-face.

"How 'bout I schedule to meet with him when I actually have a question or concern?"

"No can do. We've been doing this a long time, Terri. You may not feel like you're going to need to talk with him on a weekly basis now, and maybe not even in the first couple weeks of your treatment, but it's good to know you have a date reserved in the event something does crop up."

"Makes sense, I suppose. So I'll see you on Monday for my dry run. Thanks for the schedule."

"You're welcome. That's my phone number on the top right corner. Call me or the general office number if you have any questions."

"I will. Thanks."

Chapter 27

Mapping. Check. Another task completed on my Kick Cancer to the Curb campaign. I drove back to the office following the route I'd be taking to and from the Cancer Center on days when my session landed during a work day. I wanted to calculate exactly how much time I'd need to allocate, to avoid missing my precious time slot.

I pulled into the office parking lot. *Fifteen minutes. Add in another five to undress when I get to the hospital, five for the zapping, five to re-dress, and 15 back to the office. Forty-five minutes tip-to-finish. If nothing goes wrong. No pressure.*

"Thanks for covering the switchboard for me, Marie."

"You're welcome. How'd everything go?"

"Aside from the fact that my upper body looks something like a cross between a blueprint, a side of beef, and a Simplicity 101 dress pattern, not too bad."

"You got drawn on? Is it permanent?"

"Semi. They tell me the black ink will eventually wear off, but the tattoos are mine to keep."

"Tattoos?"

"It's a long story. I'll fill you in later. Thanks again for covering."

"No prob."

My primary function as a receptionist was to answer the switchboard, but there were also a handful of other tasks that I performed, some of which could be done after-hours. I asked Helen if I could make up my lost time at the end of each day so I wouldn't have to dip into my vacation time. She resisted a little, afraid that I'd be too tired to tack on another 30 to 45 minutes.

"Didn't you tell me that one of the side-effects of radiation is fatigue?" Helen asked.

"I did. I'm a pretty tough cookie, though. I'm banking on plowing through full speed ahead." *Please say yes. This is not how I want to use up my vacation time.*

"Okay, we can give it a try. But I'm going to be watching you." She made that gesture of two fingers pointing to her eyes, then with a turn of the wrist, pointing to my eyes.

"Honestly, you're such a mother hen!"

"I care about you. You're not just an employee, you're my friend. I'm so proud of you." She looked like she was going to cry.

"Proud?"

"You've handled this whole ordeal with such grace. I don't think I'd have even an ounce of your strength if I had cancer."

"Yes, you would. I'm nothing special. If anything, I'm just plain lucky."

"Getting cancer doesn't sound lucky to me," Helen said.

Embarrassed. Guilty. How do those words sound?

I thanked God every day that technology found my cancer early, but there were times when I was downright embarrassed to share my story with other survivors. My battle was lightweight compared to theirs. To fight Stage IV cancer you needed a bazooka, while you could get by with a water pistol or maybe even a slingshot to face off with a Stage I diagnosis like mine. Escaping the need for chemotherapy, I still had a full head of hair. My lumpectomy left me with two breasts, albeit missmatched, but I still had the full set. Aside from a boat-load of emotional battery, piles of paperwork, and a five-digit hit to our finances, I was sitting pretty. In the world of the pink ribbon, weaving five or six weeks of radiation treatments into my schedule was nothing. I got lucky. I knew it. But it wasn't anything to feel proud about.

The office grapevine spread the news of my upcoming daily radiation. I got a lot of hugs, concerned faces, and a ton of "if-there's-anything-I-can-do-just-asks" from my co-workers. Marie assured me it would be no problem to cover the switchboard, and she seemed genuinely sincere. It still killed me, though, to have to depend on her. I hated feeling indebted. Cancer was a big enough pain in *my* butt; I didn't want it to be a pain in anyone else's.

Dress Rehearsal Monday. I left my house at 7:10 a.m. to arrive at the Cancer Center by 7:35. A simple wave to Tina at the check-in desk was all I needed; her computerized masterpiece of a schedule already told her who I was. The next stop was the changing room where I quickly ripped off my clothes (waist-up) and jewelry, and wrapped myself in a heavy, warm, terrycloth robe. *Hmm, terrycloth. Nice touch. No paper gowns in this center! I wonder what* that's *costing me?* Seven-forty-five. *BAM! Right on time.*

I made my way to the waiting area, and I was almost immediately greeted by a too-cheerful-for-seven-forty-five-a.m. tech. "Good Morning," she sang. "Remember me? LeeAnn. I did your mapping."

Wow. They really do run the stopwatch here.

"I do remember. Love my tattoos, by the way."

"How are you doing this morning?"

"A little nervous. I think I'm more anxious about how this affects my work schedule than anything."

"I know it's a big time commitment. We'll do our best to get you in and out. Let's get started."

LeeAnn ushered me to the radiation room, where I was introduced to another tech named Brian. She explained that although the staff could change from day to day, there would always be two technicians giving me my treatment. Brian seemed nice enough, although a part of me (the breast part of me) always felt slightly uncomfortable when a male nurse, tech, or doctor was involved in my case. I knew they were professionals, but it still felt weird having any man other than Ludwig touching my breasts, or even looking at them. Fixing a malfunctioning arm or a leg was one thing. Analyzing and manipulating my "girls" was altogether different.

George Clooney in a white coat? Now that'd be a different story.

"If you'd step behind that curtain, Terri, and remove your robe, there's a pillowcase for you to hold across your chest. LeeAnn and I'll meet you at the exam table."

What's up with the pillowcases? Seems kind of primitive. Maybe I'll ask.

When I came out from behind the curtain, Brian and LeeAnn were on either side of the narrow table, which was dressed in crisp white cotton. *Again, no paper. Nice.* My custom-made plasti-pillow awaited my arrival. I climbed aboard, holding on to the pillowcase and my modesty with a tight grip. As I reclined, LeeAnn instinctively held my cover-up in place, while Brian guided my arms over my head and into the hollows of the plastic form. *Yeah, this is my pillow. A little hard, but mine. A perfect fit.*

Brian and LeeAnn went about calibrating their equipment, shifting my upper body ever so slightly, to the right, left, a tad more to the left, like a wad of wet clay, molding me until I was positioned just right. Dr. Gates entered the staging area, I'm not sure why—the techs seemed to be doing all the work. He showed his approval with a lot of *uh-huh's* and *looks good's.* After the final act, he'd get all the applause, and the stage hands would have nothing but the clean-up to remind them of their contributions. Two minutes later, he whooshed out the door, on to his next curtain call.

"Looks like we're all set," LeeAnn said. "We'll see you tomorrow for your first official treatment. Do you have any questions?"

This would be the perfect time to ask about the pillowcases. Nah. Why take away the intrigue?

Chapter 28

As I was driving to my first treatment, my cell phone rang. *Damn. Who could be calling me this early in the morning?* Ellie.

"Hi, Mom."

"Hi, honey. What are you doing up so early? I thought you students slept until noon every day."

"Very funny. Can you talk?"

Why now? This is the worst time to talk! "Of course I can talk. What's up? Now you're scaring me."

"Last night Josh told me his mom has breast cancer again. And I guess it's worse than last time."

"No way. She's been cancer-free for how many years? Ten?"

"Thirteen. Josh and I were in third grade at Merton."

"What do you mean by 'it's worse this time?'"

"I don't get it completely. Josh said something about it's not contained in one area—the cancer's showing up in kind of a 'fingering pattern' and they're not sure how far or where it's traveled."

"Did she have a mastectomy the first time?"

"I never knew for sure, but I think it might be on the other side now. She's gonna need chemo again, *and* radiation, and probably a lot of surgery."

"Oh my God, Ellie. That's awful. How's Josh?"

"Terrible. You know how close he and his mom are."

"Thanks for letting me know. Call me when you know more details, especially about her treatment . . . and what they're saying her prognosis is."

"I will."

"Think positive. She's so much stronger than she was thirteen years ago. My God, she turned herself into an Ironwoman! I don't know of any woman stronger, physically or mentally, than Sue."

"I know. That's what makes it so frustrating. How can she be so healthy and fit and still get cancer? Again!"

"Beats me. Why did I get cancer? Why does anyone? Let's talk later, okay? I really have to go."

"Okay. Thanks for listening. Are you on your way to work?"

"I have a stop to make on the way, then work. Love you."

"Love you, too."

Ellie didn't ask what my stop was, and I didn't offer. She didn't remember that this morning was my first radiation treatment. I knew I told her the date at some point, but it's not a detail she'd typically store in her memory bank. Ludwig and I have always had a "call us any time, day or night" policy with the kids. She didn't realize how lousy her timing was, sharing such painful news on the first day I finally felt a tiny smidge of empowerment toward fighting my cancer. And I wasn't going to tell her. A mom knows when her kid is hurting, even when that kid is 70 miles away. I sensed Ellie needed to unload her pain, and as deflated and sad as I felt after hearing her news, I silently added the weight of her sadness to mine.

I was still a good 10 minutes away from pulling into the parking lot, and my head was spinning as I fought back anger and tears.

Don't be late.
Sue's got cancer again.
Why did I wear so much jewelry today?
Cancer hit her twice!
Red light.
Shit!
Good time to take off my jewelry.
Can't be late.
Friggin' cancer.
There's no outrunning it.
Sue's a marathoner and couldn't outrun it.
It's bigger than we are. Bigger and faster.
Who are we kidding?
Green light.

"Move it!" I shouted at the car in front of me.

I took the stairs two at a time, waved my arrival to Tina, changed into a robe, and plunked down in the waiting area, a full three minutes ahead of schedule. *It helped taking the jewelry off in the car.* I finally had time to let go of my tears. *How could Sue have cancer again?*

"Gooood morning, Terri."
What? Can you not see that I'm crying?
"Morning, LeeAnn."

"So are you excited to get started with your treatment?"

"Not so much."

LeeAnn looked confused, almost hurt, like I was being a party-pooper.

"Oh? What's up? You look upset." We walked to the zapping room.

"I just found out a friend of mine's been re-diagnosed with breast cancer after thirteen years clean. Thirteen years."

"Why don't you change out of your robe, Terri. We'll talk at the table."

I cooperated, even though at that moment I honestly didn't feel I had a rat's ass chance in hell that I was ever going to be completely free from cancer. It was all smoke and mirrors—surgery, radiation, oncologists. A giant farce. A billion-dollar industry tied up with a pretty pink ribbon.

More tears.

Just like yesterday, Brian and LeeAnn stood on their imaginary X's on opposite sides of the table, waiting to perform their "miracles." They were starting to look less like people to me and more like robots standing at attention in their faded-from-too-many-washings scrubs.

"You remember Brian?" LeeAnn asked.

"I do."

I climbed onto the table and Brian helped me get situated into my plastic pillow.

"So tell me about your friend," LeeAnn said.

"Sue. She's the mother of my daughter's friend, Josh. She and I aren't terribly close, but Ellie's known Josh since kindergarten, so there's definitely a history."

"And how old are Ellie and Josh now?"

"They're both twenty-one. They met on the school bus sixteen years ago, and they're still in school together at UW Madison."

I caught Brian glancing at the clock, not at all interested in joining our chick-chat. I could see it in his eyes: "Come on, LeeAnn. Focus."

She must have missed his nonverbal cue, because she invited him in. "Terri was just telling me about a friend of hers who was just diagnosed with breast cancer."

I noticed a tiny vein pulsating in his temple and emphasized, "Re-diagnosed. She's been cancer-free for thirteen years. What d'ya know. Bam! It found her again." I looked directly at Brian. "Explain *that*."

His temple-vein became more pronounced. "As much as I'd like to, I *can't* explain it," Brian said. "All we can do is not admit defeat. Science and technology have come too far to quit now. We can't give up on the hope for a cure."

"Bad answer. No offense, but from my perspective it's looking more and more like we're all chasing our tails trying to look busy and not really getting anywhere. Cancer still wins. What's the point in going through any of this?" I pointed with my nose to the bulky machinery hanging over my torso.

Code Red. Code Red. Patient turning hostile.

Robots 1 and 2 tried to come across as unaffected, but I sensed the tiniest chink in their demeanors as soon as I started finding fault with their answers. They continued systematically adjusting the supposed cancer-killing machines *(HA! They're probably stage props)*, each of them waiting for the other to come up with a suitable response to my negative and combative attitude.

Brian drew the short straw. "The point of going through this is that we have to address what we know now. To not treat your cancer now because you think you might get cancer in the future just doesn't make sense. You may be lucky enough to *never* get cancer again."

"Oh, so it comes down to luck. How scientific!"

LeeAnn came to his rescue. "Your friend lived thirteen more years because of the treatment she received. Not everyone is that lucky."

I spat back, "And now Lady Luck is about to lose all her hair, probably both breasts, and maybe her life."

Brian and LeeAnn looked at each other with blank stares, speechless.

I gave them their out. "Thanks for trying, but this conversation isn't going to end on a positive note. I know we have to stay on schedule. Whatever. Let's continue going through the motions. Zap me."

LeeAnn gently smoothed my pillowcase before retreating to the safety of the radiation-free "gool" behind the thick pane of glass. Brian followed, checking his watch, probably wondering how and why he got sucked into the chick-chat in the first place.

And I lay still and vulnerable beneath the cancer-killing machine *(right)*, tears slowly making their way down toward my ears, landing with the tiniest of taps onto my custom-made, hard, plastic pillow.

Lucky me.

Chapter 29

The first few weeks of radiation were fairly uneventful. I had the timing of driving the route to the Cancer Center down to a science, fully aware of where the cops hung out, which lanes plugged up with morning slow-pokes, and which intersections to use to never get caught at a red light. Admittedly, I took a few liberties relative to the rules of the road, and I always made sure my radiation schedule was conveniently placed on the front passenger seat next to me to show the small-town fuzz that I was a "poor victim of cancer, just trying to get to my radiation treatment on time." I'd rehearse my sob-story into my rearview mirror (*sniff*), then break out laughing at how gutsy it would be to actually use it as my defense if I got pulled over for racing through an amber or rolling a stop sign.

End-of-the-day fatigue didn't start to surface until week three, and the browning of my breast and area surrounding my armpit began shortly after that. The next probable side effect would be burning and sometimes peeling of the skin, and I was strongly encouraged by Dr. Gates (although I fought it as long as I could) to switch from my normal antiperspirant to an aluminum-free deodorant before that happened.

Deodorant does NOT prevent wetness, and of course the recommended brand was unscented, so between potentially walking around the office with dark sweat rings under my pits and smelling like a pre-pubescent 12-year old, I stubbornly took the chance and stuck to my Summer-Breeze Ban Roll-on. Then I burned. And peeled. And finally gave in to the crappy-doctor-recommended-useless-unscented-deodorant.

The plan to make up my daily lost time from the office at the end of each day worked out pretty well. Helen was all over me to go home if I felt tired, but anyone who's muscled their way through raising babies knows how to push fatigue aside when it's not welcome. Getting a daily dose of radiation paled in comparison to the months of sleep deprivation I went through when Ellie and Karl were babies. I tried to squeeze in a few visits to the gym each week, but working out was no longer a priority in my life, at least not until I could slather my pits with an authentic antiperspirant of my choice!

My spirit was still somewhat bruised throughout my treatment. In my deepest heart I knew the right thing to do was to fight my cancer, despite my ever-present skepticism and doubt that treatment would insulate me from a re-diagnosis. I held on to the fantasy that the team of medical pros on my bench really did want to cure me and were not part of a conspiracy to use my disease to fund their exotic vacation destinations or pay for their children's Ivy League college educations. I had so many friends praying for and believing in my recovery that it just didn't feel right to shoot down their devotion, however naïve their hope seemed to be.

"Kill 'em. Kill 'em." There were days when I'd lie on the table and quietly whisper the words over and over, as the radiation penetrated what remained of my breast. I imagined cancer cells popping in tiny explosions, burning to a crisp in puffs of white smoke. A handful of radiation techs, including LeeAnn and Brian, administered my treatments, and all were consistently professional and positive. Dr. Gates and I met for a few minutes every Monday, but I never took too much away from those appointments. He seemed more concerned with what kind of deodorant I was using than anything else.

One week I was so fed up with him obsessing about the deodorant issue that I beat him to the punch. "Please, Dr. Gates. If you're going to ask me if I'm using the recommended aluminum-free deodorant instead of my antiperspirant, I'm going to have to leave this room right now. We cannot have that conversation again!"

He looked at me like I just kicked him in the groin, and said, "So noted."

Between the expression on his face and his simple, two-word response, "so noted," I couldn't remember the last time I laughed that hard or long. For the first time in months, I felt like I was in control. Control of the White Coats, my cancer, my future.

Dr. Gates patiently waited for me to regain my composure. "Well then, I guess I'll see you next Monday." He still looked confused and befuddled.

Holding back another round of hysterics, I managed to politely answer, "Yes, I guess you will."

That laugh carried me for weeks.

Chapter 30

As I was coming to the end of my radiation treatments, Dr. Gates reminded me that I still needed to meet with a medical oncologist. One more doctor to add to my team roster. The bench was looking a little lonely, anyway. When I was first diagnosed, there were all kinds of medical professionals and cheerleaders shaking their pompoms on my behalf. I thought they'd have my back through my whole treatment journey. Boy, was I mistaken. That's not at all how it works. The pros kind of rotate in, like pinch hitters, do their thing, then move on to the next game. It's not that they're not dedicated, it's just that with one-in-eight women getting hit with breast cancer, there's always a new lump in someone's road that needs blasting. Sad but true, cancer is a supply-and-demand, billion-dollar industry with a shelf-life as long as a Hostess Twinkie. Cancer keeps a lot of people employed, including funeral directors.

"Okay . . . tell me again what the medical oncologist does?" *Is he the butcher, the baker, or the candlestick maker?*

Dr. Gates patiently answered, "The medical oncologist specializes in treating cancer through drug therapy."

"Oh, I remember. Drugs are the third phase of my treatment plan: surgery, radiation, drug therapy."

"That's right. A common regimen for your type of breast cancer is that you take an estrogen receptor like Tamoxifen, for example."

"Estrogen receptor? Tamoxifen?" *Sounds like a prehistoric dinosaur: Tamoxi-fena-saurus.*

"Your oncologist will explain everything in more detail. There are quite a lot of different theories and research findings to weigh before choosing which, if any, drug therapy option is right for you."

"How long would I have to stay on the drug?"

"Five years is the standard, but again, there are a lot of factors that come into play and various options to explore and consider. It's not my area of expertise."

Yeah, you already said that. No need to squirm in your undershorts, Dr. Gates. I'm not recording our conversation.

"One last question. Where can I find one of those miracle, HA!, I mean *medical* oncologists?" *How does he keep such a straight face?*

"Our Center has two doctors that I'd highly recommend, Dr. Richards and Dr. Mertin. You'd start with a consultation. It's a good idea to bring another set of ears along, like your husband or a friend—there's a lot of information to digest. Look for an appointment any time within the next couple of weeks."

"Sorry. I guess I have one more question. Do I finish my radiation therapy before I start with the drugs?"

"You do. Typically there's about a one-month gap between the two therapies. Any more questions?"

That depends if you're being sincere or sarcastic.

"Not off the top of my head. Looks like I'd better get moving on setting up a consult. I think I've only got about fifteen more treatments left with you. Where *does* the time go?"

That one got a little chuckle out of Dr. Gates. Although he still wasn't exactly on my A-List, we were starting to find a certain rhythm with one another. I think the crack I made about deodorant a couple of weeks ago knocked him out of his auto-pilot mode. He didn't dump my case onto any of his colleagues, so I assumed he was still okay with taking my money. I guess doctors have a pretty high tolerance for patients who are vocal.

Chapter 31

After reading the biographies of both of the medical oncologists that Dr. Gates recommended, I was leaning toward Dr. Richards. I'd grown somewhat chummy with some of the Center's staff, so I picked their brains as to which doc they would choose if they were undergoing treatment. They're always extremely careful to not incriminate themselves by sharing their opinions about the White Coats, but I'd learned how to decode their whispered, round-about responses: "Wink, wink, if you know what I mean, you didn't hear it from me," usually meant to steer clear. "Don't quote me, but there's a reason you can't get on his book," meant he was the crowd favorite.

Both doctors seemed like good choices, but Dr. Richards was my pick. *Would have been better if the doc was a she, not a he, but no such luck.* A rare opening emerged on his calendar due to a cancellation, so I snatched the spot quicker than a kid grabbing the last seat in a game of Musical Chairs. I took a chance that Ludwig would be able to join me for the consultation—he was getting used to having to drop-and-go, and if he was feeling any push-back from his boss, I didn't know about it. Honestly, who would deny a guy the right to hold his wife's hand through her cancer treatment? *Ebeneezer Scrooge comes to mind.*

Ludwig and I sat down with Dr. Richards and added yet another tier of facts and statistics to our already teetering Jenga tower of cancer information. His approach to educating us was organized and direct, which appealed to Ludwig, but the doc didn't come across like he was reciting his lines by rote for the umpteenth time, which earned him a gold star from me. He was just the right blend of professor and grandfather. Bill Nye the Science Guy and Mr. Rogers. The perfect closer to see me through the last leg of my journey.

The drug therapy phase of my treatment was the most technical and difficult to comprehend. Despite Dr. Richards' attempt to explain the process in simple terms, it didn't take long before his words started spinning like pieces of fruit in a smoothie blender. It would have been nice to have Ellie and her biology-brains in the room with us to help us wade through the quagmire of technical terms and concepts. At one point I wondered, *is he even speaking in English?*

Dr. Richards took a breath and looked at both of us. "Are you following this?"

I fessed up. "Sort of. Well, not exactly. No. Okay, not even a little."

The horizontal lines in Ludwig's forehead were more pronounced than usual. My guess was that he was just as lost as I was.

I asked him, "You getting any of this, Ludwig? Or am I the only one in the room wearing a dunce cap?"

"I was on track about a quarter of the way, then I got lost, too. Can you start again, Dr. Richards?"

"No problem. The more you chew on this stuff, the easier it starts to go down."

"Well, I'm ready for seconds, but I'll take mine pureed this time."

Dr. Richards chuckled, "Good to hear you have a sense of humor, Terri."

"You haven't heard the last of it," Ludwig jumped in. "Trust me, she's got a whole collection of one-liners in her grab-bag. Once she flips her switch, there's no going back."

"Hello . . . I'm in the room, Ludwig. I can hear you!"

"Okay, then. Let's start over. Tamoxifen is a prescription medication that is like estrogen in some ways and different in others. In the breast, it can block estrogen's effects."

"That's where you lost me. Estrogen's effects?" I asked.

"Cancers like yours, that are estrogen- or progesterone-receptor positive, need estrogen to grow."

"So the Tamoxifen blocks the estrogen to prevent that growth?"

"That's the goal, but there are no guarantees. It *may* prevent the growth of future breast cancer cells, *may* being the operative word."

"It's a crapshoot."

"I wouldn't call it a crapshoot." He whipped out a notepad from his coat pocket and started scribbling down statistics.

"A U.S. study looked at women with your type of cancer and compared those who took Tamoxifen for five years with others who took a placebo. Out of every one thousand women who took the drug, each year about ten got breast cancer. Out of every one thousand women who took the placebo, about seventeen got cancer."

Ludwig, the human calculator, chimed in, "That means one percent of the drug women got cancer versus one-point-seven percent of the placebo women. That's not much of a difference—point seven percent. I would have thought there'd be a wider spread between the two."

I added, "You're right. Ten versus seventeen. Ten women still got cancer, with or without the drug—that's a wash. It's the other seven that got stuck with the placebo that got screwed, pardon my French. Seven isn't such a big number when you compare it to one thousand. It's big only if you're one of the seven."

The room got quiet.

"I'm guessing there are side effects?"

"With any medication, there are potential side effects and risk factors, which is why some women forego taking the drug. You have to be comfortable with the benefits versus risk-and-side-effect ratio."

I mumbled under my breath, "It can never be easy."

"Pardon?"

"I said, it can never be easy. Every decision we've had to make since the damned shadow showed up on my mammogram eight months ago has been difficult. Why can it never, never be easy?" My sense of humor went into hiding.

"I wish I had an answer for you . . . an easy answer . . . but I don't. Cancer is complicated."

"I apologize for my sudden mood change. I don't mean to sound disrespectful. It's just so frustrating having to make these decisions and never quite feeling qualified to make them. No offense, but the medical professionals who have the knowledge don't seem willing to make the decisions—it always comes down to us. The ones without the medical degrees. It's frustrating."

"As doctors, we can only present options from a medical standpoint. There are countless other factors that come into play that reach beyond medicine . . . a whole sphere that makes your world yours. You know that world better than anyone."

A decent attempt at rebuttal. Practiced (Bill Nye), with a touch of compassion (Mr. Rogers).

"Should I continue with the potential side effects?" Dr. Richards asked.

"Fire away. We're all ears."

"I'm not going to lie, the list is long. Everything from hot flashes to blood clots, stroke, liver problems. Cataracts. Will you experience any of these? You may or may not."

"There's that operative word again. *May.*"

"Or may not," Dr. Richards added.

"And I'd have to take it for how long? Five years?"

"Studies show there are no additional benefits to taking the medication for longer than five years."

"Could I try it out on a trial basis to see if I experience any side effects?"

"Absolutely."

"Because if I have a stroke or go blind, I'm gonna stop taking it!"

"Sounds fair."

"Am I monitored in some way to see if the drug is hammering away at any of my innards without me knowing it?"

"I'll see you on an annual basis for a series of blood tests and analyses. Do you think you can tolerate me once a year, Terri?"

"Oh, now I've gone and hurt your feelings, Dr. Richards. You're kidding me, right?"

"I am. Doctors have senses of humor, too, you know."

"Touchè!"

"Go home and think it over. You've got at least a month-and-a-half before you'd even start the drug therapy phase. You and your husband don't have to make a decision now."

Ludwig stood, extending his hand. "That sounds good, Dr. Richards. Thanks for your time."

"You're welcome. I'll walk you out and get some reading material for you to take home. My card will be attached. Call me if you have any questions. You're almost done with your radiation, Terri. Stay positive. You're moving in the right direction. Forward."

"Forward's better than backward, I guess. Unless there's a pile of dog . . ." Ludwig stopped me before I could finish my sentence. "Okay, then. We'll be in touch. Thanks, again."

I held back a tsunami of laughter as Ludwig and I hustled down the flight of stairs and out of the building. It wasn't just the impending reference to dog doo-doo that was behind the wave. It was more the simple need to release all the tension and frustration building up inside of me. As soon as we hit the parking lot, I exploded into a wave of laughter, followed by a second wave of tears. The tide of my conflicting emotions ebbed and flowed, and Ludwig sheltered me as best he could, silently holding me in his arms.

Chapter 32

In my final two weeks of radiation, I was scheduled to receive three "booster treatments." Along with the normal doses of radiation, I'd get an additional, more concentrated dose aimed directly at the spot where my tumor had been removed. As if my skin weren't tender and burnt enough, they planned on cranking up the heat a few more notches from simmer to boil, just for good measure. A cancer cell would have to be quite a hard-ass to survive a beating like that.

Boost away, but if I smell smoke, I'm bailing.

Beginning each and every day trekking out to the cancer center was starting to get old. Only a handful of my co-workers even remembered I was still in treatment, and routinely asked how I was doing. But for the rest, my cancer seemed to be yesterday's news. One of my life observations is that the stronger you are (or appear to be), the more alone you are. Sure, when I first made the announcement to the office that I had breast cancer, there were all kinds of hugs and tears, and offers to "help in any way I can . . . really, Terri. Anything you need, just ask." People mean well. But it's more common than not to put the burden of asking for help on the one who's hurting instead of taking the initiative of offering help without being asked.

Getting zapped with radiation wasn't terribly painful. The morning race to the cancer center, the undressing, the techs' cold hands on my naked skin, the noise from the machine, the having to lie perfectly still, the re-dressing, the speeding back to work. All the while wondering whether absorbing a poison like radiation in order to kill a poison like cancer was doing my body more harm than good. That's what made the daily procedure painful. Hearing the words from a co-worker, "Let me drive you tomorrow. We'll stop for coffee on the way back to the office," would have meant so much. But the strength I wore on my face let everyone off the hook. I guess the loneliness I felt was *my* fault. After all, I didn't ask. What did I expect?

More.

Chapter 33

Some dates are forever stamped in my memory. June 24, 2011 is one of those dates. The red circle around the 24th marked the 33rd, and last, day of my radiation. Graduation Day. Liberation Day. *"In Your Face, Cancer!"* Day. My car radio blared as I pulled into the cancer center parking lot. I took the stairs two at a time, and when I reached the second floor I spotted my surgeon in the corridor.

"Good morning, Dr. Gallos!"

"Good morning," she replied politely, but I could tell she didn't have a clue who I was—I'd put money on it. Now if I'd lifted up my blouse and showed her my scars, that would've been a different story. *"Ah, Case No. 43997. I remember you. Stage I. Tiny tumor. Clean lymph nodes."* Normally I would have been offended that a doctor who took a scalpel to my breast just four-and-a-half months ago didn't have the decency to remember me, but nothing was going to ruin my red-circle day. Not even a doctor's indifference.

Yeah, whatever. Have a nice day, doc.

Like so many mornings before this one, I proceeded to the changing room and threw on a terrycloth robe, which felt surprisingly soft this morning. *My last treatment and they finally found the fabric softener!* The crème de la crème of my red-circle day though, was that my two favorite techs were on duty to fire off the last round of ammo at my withered, what-in-the-heck-is-that-thing? breast.

"Hi, Terri. Congratulations! Number 33. You made it," LeeAnn sang cheerfully.

"I did. Today's my grand finale. After today you two won't have *me* to push around anymore."

Brian answered, "That's okay with us. As far as we're concerned, we don't ever want to see you here again!"

"Well, that's a fine how-do-you-do," I said with a laugh.

"I told you thirty-three treatments ago that's how I'd send you off. I wasn't lying," said LeeAnn. "All kidding aside, this really is a special day. We're so proud of you."

"Now stop that, you guys. You're going to make me cry."

"We allow crying, as long as they're happy tears," said LeeAnn.

"The compassion you two have shown has helped make this nightmare bearable. Angels. You both should be wearing gossamer wings and halos."

LeeAnn laughed, "Stop. Picturing Brian in that get-up . . . now you're making *me* cry. Brian, are you blushing?"

"Let's say we get Terri on the table so she can get outta' here. I swear . . ." Brian trailed off, shaking his head.

LeeAnn answered in an exaggerated whisper, "All business, that Brian. We've got a little something special to give you on your way out. Don't let me forget."

"Hmmm. Does it have leather or cloth interior? I'd prefer leather. Can I choose?"

"HA! Nothing quite as elaborate as that, not that you don't deserve it."

I hopped onto the table and nestled into my customized plastic pillow. *I wonder if I get to take this home with me. It wouldn't fit anyone else, and I did pay for it. Dearly.* My senses were amplified as I lay back, ready to soak in my last doses of radiation. The noise from the machine, the temperature of the room, the bright red laser beams marking their target: it was all more vivid today. I closed my eyes, and a reel of film flickered flashbacks of the past few months through my mind—*It's cancer . . . Ludwig, can you come to the hospital? . . . Early, we found it early . . . You're a lucky woman . . . Hey kids, it's mom . . . Don't worry, it's beatable . . . Lucky woman—it didn't spread . . . Lumpectomy . . . Radiation . . . It's cancer. . . Are you sure you got it all? . . . Will I ever be sure? . . . Ever?*

"Terri? Terri, we're done." The sound of Brian's voice brought me back into the room. The tail of the film strip wound down, a staccato click, click, click, a blur of black and white snips, then nothing.

"Are you okay?" LeeAnn helped me sit up. She noticed I'd been crying. "Let me get those tears." She snatched a tissue from a side table and gently dabbed my temples in a final display of angelic compassion.

"I'm fine. I guess the emotions are running at full tilt this morning."

"That's perfectly okay. Let's get you on your way. Oh, I almost forgot your surprise."

"Cloth seats are fine. Really."

No car. *Oh well.* Instead, LeeAnn handed me a Certificate of Completion, signed by all the technicians, with little scrawled messages of hope: "You go girl!" "Nice work!" "You beat it!" "Way to go!"

Way better than a car. A Certificate of Completion. Take that, cancer! Don't you ever show your ugly face in my life again.

LeeAnn and I shared a final round of hugs (Brian held back and offered a friendly handshake), and I danced off to the changing room to slam dunk my robe into the hamper for the last time. In the privacy of the dressing room I re-read the handwritten messages, but I noticed the absence of Dr. Gates' name.

No surprise. The great divide between technicians and doctors. Whatever.

"Who's that singing in there?" The voice, tiny as it was, caught me off guard. I thought I was alone.

How embarrassing. I hope I was singing on key.

I cracked open the door of my dressing room, poking my head out like a turtle from under its shell. The little voice came from an equally little woman, who was sitting in the waiting room. The first thing I noticed was how disproportionately big her terrycloth robe looked on her tiny frame, as though she had jumped feet-first into a snow drift. All that peeked out was her head, which was wrapped in a scarf, a futile attempt to cover her baldness.

Damn. That little lady has cancer.

I skipped putting on my jewelry, quickly shoved my robe deep into the hamper, and left my changing room. I didn't want to risk not being able to meet the talking snow drift.

"It was me," I answered. "Hi, my name is Terri."

"Hi, Terri. I'm Nora."

She fished her boney hand out of her sleeve to offer a handshake. My guess was that Nora was in her late 60s, early 70s. It was hard to say. Chemo can age a person prematurely. No eyebrows, no eyelashes. Her pallid skin hung loose from sharply angled cheekbones. Skin and bones.

"Nice to meet you, Nora." I sat next to her on the loveseat.

"Tell me, Terri, what's put such a song in your heart this morning?" Nora's smile revealed a full set of brilliant white dentures, too big for her shrunken mouth. (They clicked when she talked.)

"I just had my last radiation treatment. I'm done, well-done, fried to a crisp."

"Oh, that's wonderful! Not that you're fried to a crisp, that you're done with your treatment. Show me your diploma." She noticed the certificate in my hands.

My heart was breaking as I shared my certificate with her. We were locked together in the same minute of time, but each of our minutes was so different. I had broken free from cancer—she was still restrained in its embrace.

"How far along are you in your treatment, Nora?"

"I have just five more chemotherapy treatments, then I start my radiation. It's been a long haul this time around, what with my Bill gone almost three years now, but I'm trying to stay positive."

"This time?"

"This is number two for me. They took one of my breasts the first time, back in eighty-one. And wouldn't you know, cancer goes and finds my other breast thirty years later. Big appetite, that cancer." Nora laughed at her own witty candidness.

I couldn't hold back my tears. "I'm sorry you have to go through this again. It's so unfair."

Nora took my hand in hers. "I don't know how old you are, Terri, but I'm guessing you're old enough to know that fair's got nothing to do with it. I got through it once. I'll get through it again. That's what we do."

"Get through it?"

"That's right. We get through it."

Nora gave my hand a little pat and said, "Now be happy, dang it! Get that song back in your heart and get the heck out of here. You're a beautiful young woman. This is your day to be happy. You worked hard for it. Mine'll come in no time. These old bones got a lot of livin' left in them."

"I'll be praying for you, Nora. You take care."

I did get out of there, but the song in my heart was replaced with a one-syllable, angry roar. I couldn't shake Nora's image from my mind, the tiny, bald woman drowning in the big white robe. Skin and bones. How could I take a victory lap knowing Nora, and thousands of others, were still at the starting line?

Some would never even see the finish line, much less cross it. Not everyone was as lucky as I was.

I drove the familiar route from the Center to my office through a blur of tears, ranting, "It's not fair, it's just not fair." I didn't care how accepting Nora seemed to be with her diagnosis. By the time you hit your 70s, you should be able to finally sit back and take in all the sights. "With a full head of hair and matching eyebrows!" I shouted into my rearview mirror. You shouldn't have to drag yourself to a cancer center every day to be manhandled by strangers in white coats and pastel scrubs. Tossing your guts into a toilet should come only from sprinkling too much paprika into your stew, not from a round of chemo coursing through your veins.

I sat in the hot silence of my car in my office parking lot, drained, my cheeks salt-stained from crying. I stared at my Certificate of Completion, re-reading the cheerful sentiments: "Nice work!" "You beat it!"

Will Nora? It isn't fair. It's just not fair.

Chapter 34

My other life—my non-cancer life—was waiting for me to turn on the lights, open the switch-board, and put on a happy face. I recited my phone greeting as I dragged myself up the two flights of stairs to the office:

Good morning! How may I direct your call?

Good morning! Thank you for calling. How may I direct you?

Good morning! Life isn't fair. How may I direct you?

Good morning! Cancer is bigger than we are. When are we going to admit it?

I still had 10 minutes to burn before show time, so I headed for the break room, hoping one of the early arrivals had started a pot of coffee. The rich aroma of a fresh brew placed its warm hand on my shoulder—just what I needed to rewind and restart the morning on a more positive track. One of my favorite young agents was preparing his cup for his first pour of the day.

"Morning, Joe."

"Hey, Terri. You're in luck. The pot's almost ready."

"That, my friend, is music to my ears."

"Why's that? Bad night?"

"Bad morning."

Joe stopped what he was doing and gave me his full attention, which was all it took for me to break down and cry again. He kept the space between us, but looked directly at me. Eye contact was one of Joe's best assets—once he made the commitment to engage in a conversation with you, he'd lock the door with his eyes, and distractions were not allowed in, no matter how hard they knocked.

"What's going on?" he asked.

"This morning was my last radiation treatment. Number 33. All done."

"That's great news. Why the tears?"

"While I was jumping for joy getting ready to leave the Center, I met the sweetest old lady in the dressing room. Nora. I'm guessing she was around seventy. Completely bald. She was waiting to get her chemo treatment. She told me this was her second bout with cancer."

"That stinks," Joe said. If my crying made him uncomfortable, he hung tough. He didn't look away.

"I feel so guilty and ashamed."

"Why ashamed?"

"Because I got off so easy. No chemo. No bald head. A little lumpectomy and a month-and-a-half of radiation, and I'm good to go."

Joe broke the invisible, politically correct barrier and gave me a hug, quick but sincere.

"How can you even say you got off easy? None of what you went through had to have been easy. They found your cancer early, right? You shouldn't feel guilty *or* ashamed."

"Yeah, cancer shouldn't pick on sweet old ladies like Nora. I hate how it feasts on weak and easy targets. I'm younger and stronger. I could have taken more."

"So finishing your treatment is bittersweet. I still don't think you should feel guilty. I'm gonna be happy you're done. Now, can I pour you a mug?"

"That'd be nice." We raised our cups. "To Nora."

PART 4

——

Defense

Chapter 35

Pills or no pills. One pill a day for the next five years. 1,825 pills. Once again fear nipped at my heels, chasing me into my decision. The fear of new cancer developing if I didn't medicate outweighed the fear of possible side effects from the drug if I did. Hearing the words "It's cancer" knocked most of any sense of security right out of me, but the first thing I knew for sure was that I never wanted to hear those two words again. If that meant swallowing a chemical every morning for the next five years, I'd do it. I figured it was a gamble either way; I might as well devote all my energy into kicking what I *knew* was in my path and worry about the consequences of pill-popping later. There are always consequences. That was the second thing I knew for sure.

The third thing I knew for sure was I was 30 pounds over-weight. Falling out of my regular exercise regimen and into a fairly regular habit of stress-eating probably had something to do with gaining the extra pounds. Reduced exercise plus increased food intake equals heavier object. I was that object. It's that simple. Consequences.

More challenges, please. Could I have just a few more challenges?

Coincident to my entire wardrobe shrinking like overripe grapes on a vine, an ad for an online membership to Weight Watchers popped up on my laptop one morning. Weight Watchers. Me and Weight Watchers. That was as bizarre a combo as me and breast cancer.

My ego would not allow me to jump up another clothes size, and the elastic on my granny-panties trembled precariously on their last threads, so I gave in and hit the damned "go" button, committing myself to a 90-day membership. The beauty of signing up online was the anonymity. It was humiliating enough to admit I'd gained weight—after all, I was always seen as the skinny one. Being a faceless, nameless cyberspace member also meant not being pressured by a coach to go to any of those weigh-in sessions or support group meetings I'd heard about. Having to suck in my gut to zip up my pants was demoralizing enough; admitting my lack of discipline in a room full of strangers would only intensify my embarrassment. I'd get through this setback the same way I got through seven months of cancer hell—without joining a support group!

Just like Nora said: "We get through it. That's what we do."

Once I got over the embarrassment of being in a committed relationship with a weight-loss cult, I acclimated very quickly to the method of assigning point values to the food I ate, tracking every morsel that passed through my lips, accountable to no one but my laptop. I'd never say it out loud, but it's a pretty cool system for managing out-of-control eating. Best of all, it works!

At the end of my 90-day membership I'd lost around 20 pounds, which was still 10 pounds shy of my goal. I stuck to the program on my own for another month. From June to October I lost a total of 30 pounds and dropped two whole clothes sizes, rewarding myself amply with a new and sassy wardrobe. I kicked my stretched-out bloomers to the curb, and replaced them with . . . well, that's not anything I'm going to share! It was energizing to feel in control of my health after so many months of feeling I'd been blindsided, duped, and dragged over a muddy road with an insurmountable rock in the middle of it. Friends, family, and co-workers who were not aware of my secret affair with Weight Watchers were convinced my gradual weight-loss was due to my cancer. They thought I was sick again, and my old friend Ken, from church, teared-up every Sunday after Mass, insisting my cancer was back and I was protecting him from the truth.

"You're so skinny, Terri. That's just not natural."

"Ken, I'm far from skinny."

"You're sick again. I just know it. Your cancer's back, isn't it?"

"My cancer's not back, Ken. I went on a diet, plain and simple."

"Well, I worry about you. You and Ludwig are like family."

"You've got nothing to worry about, dear friend. My cancer's not back. I'm healthier now than when I was diagnosed in January. Please, stop worrying, okay?"

Every Sunday it was the same conversation. Poor Ken. I'll never understand why people are so quick to equate weight loss with illness. As I see it, most people would be better off if they ate less and exercised more. Plain and simple.

Chapter 36

The bench was empty. For the first time in almost nine months, I was completely on my own. No more oncologists, surgeons, radiologists, or technicians. The whole roster packed their bags and left, one at a time, the last one turning off the lights. The stadium was completely empty.

Nine months ago I had breast cancer. A handful of medical professionals had come together to form a team, and they sat on my bench, each one taking their turn at bat to help me out-score the opponent. I know they were here from the footprints they left behind in the dirt, and especially from the faint brown smudge radiation left behind on my lopsided breast. I'm not sure what I expected at the end of the battle—a pizza party? Team photo? After such a long haul, the final inning felt abrupt and lonely. Just me and the scoreboard. Team Cancer: Zero. Team Terri: Won. *Yes, I did.*

But none of those pros left me with a game plan for what to do next—how to stay cancer-free. The mystery still plagues me: if we all have cancer cells in our bodies and they co-exist with healthy cells, what caused mine to suddenly begin to multiply and take over the neighborhood like a pack of playground bullies? I posed the question a dozen times during my treatment, but I never got a concrete answer, which was frustrating and puzzling. I cannot fathom (or accept) how, in the 21st century, the cause of cancer still eludes the brilliant minds of scientists. What series of events turns an otherwise healthy environment into one that becomes so attractive for the bad guys to lay down roots? I wanted to post a sign: Cancer Cells Beware. You're Not Welcome Here!

My team of medical all-stars cut and zapped the cancer right out of me, and I'll be forever grateful their expertise left me with a clean slate. I brought them cancer. They got rid of it. They did their jobs. But at the end of the road I expected more. I expected a prevention plan. A thumbs-up, a prescription for Tamoxifen, and a "Come back in six months for your follow-up mammogram," is what I got instead.

Come back in six months? Why? So we can start the whole cycle again? I just want someone to help me plan a defense. Is that asking too much?

Chapter 37

My first milestone. Five months had passed since my last radiation treatment. The standard wait-time to have a diagnostic mammogram after cancer treatment was six months, but with the holidays fast approaching, I wanted to get it over with early so I could concentrate on glad tidings and all that crap.

Ho-ho-ho and fa-la-la-la-la. Never been much of a fan.

My mammogram a year ago November was what started this whole mess. The urge to go into hiding behind the safety of a heavy door with a one-way lock was tempting, though probably not the best course of action. I pulled on my big-girl undies and scheduled the appointment.

I hate being a big girl.

The waiting room of the Breast Care Center hadn't changed one bit from a year ago. Same soft lighting. Same smell. *Lavender.* Same Ruth Ann-with-the-cute-pixie-haircut behind the desk. Coffee caddy in the corner. Handmade teddy bears with outstretched arms sat patiently on the shelf waiting to console the next woman unlucky enough to hear the words, "It's cancer." Only the dates on the magazines fanned out on the end table proved that one full year had passed.

Time to start the celestial bargaining.

Please God. No shadows this time. I promise I'll stop swearing.

And speeding.

"Hi, Terri. Remember me? Linda. Congratulations, you've come full circle!"

"Thanks, Linda. I wish I could be as excited about today as you are. I'm not going to lie. I'd rather be in the chicken line and be able to bail out right before the mammogram starts."

"You crack me up. You're a survivor, Terri. You won the battle. I can assure you this mammogram will be a yawn fest. Trust me."

I did trust her. Linda was the radiology technician who ran my mammogram last November, and because she did her job right that day, she noticed the microcalcification cluster that proved to be Stage I cancer. She was the first set of eyes on that x-ray image. Granted, there were others who reviewed the pictures she took, but I still give a lot of the credit to her for taking good images in the first place.

"Now that you've had a lumpectomy, I'll need to take a few additional images at the site of your incision. The scar tissue that develops after surgery poses a bit of a challenge on my end of the camera, so bear with me if I get a little rough."

"Thanks for the warning, but don't worry about me. Do what you have to do. Believe me, Linda, the pain of having my breast compressed as flat as an uninflated whoopy cushion is nothing compared to the panic attack I'm trying to compress in my head."

"Honestly, in all my years I've never heard anyone compare their compressed breast to a whoopy cushion. Mind if I share that with my colleagues?"

"Be my guest."

Linda proceeded to take multiple images of both breasts. She wasn't lying when she said the extra images might be painful. But pain is relative. A lumpectomy, 33 radiation treatments, and surviving a breast cancer diagnosis give new light to pain. On a pain scale of one-to-ten, the mammogram now sits at a mere three, down from an eight a year ago.

"All set, Terri. I got some really clear pictures. Anyone ever tell you you're extremely photogenic?"

"Aw, you say the nicest things."

"Have a seat in the dressing area. I'll have our radiologist, Dr. Newton, review the films. I'll come get you when she's done."

"Will do."

Please God. No new shadows. I promise I'll be more polite to the people who walk too slow in malls. And to grocery store cashiers who crack their gum.

Linda retrieved me from the dressing area a few minutes later and walked me into a dimly lit room where I could view the x-ray images with her and Dr. Newton.

Dimly lit rooms are never a good sign.

"Hi, Terri. I'm Dr. Newton. I've reviewed your mammogram images and would like to explain a few areas that concern me."

Dear God. This can't be happening. This cannot be happening.

"I'm sorry. Did you say something, Terri?"

Did I say that out loud?

158

I stared blankly at the black-and-white images clipped to the lit screens. Panic was ricocheting through my body. "Areas that concern you?"

Dr. Newton answered calmly, using the eraser end of a pencil as a wand bringing my focus to her *specific areas of concern.* "Stay with me. This first image is your mammogram from a year ago. The shadowy areas and white spots are the calcifications that we biopsied and found to be cancerous."

"Go on."

"The second image shows the temporary wires that were placed in your breast pre-surgery so Dr. Gallos would know the boundaries to follow during your lumpectomy. The wires serve as a 'map' for the surgeon to follow, so they know where and how much tissue to remove."

Dr. Newton continued waving her wand. "You can see that this area of calcification was right on the edge of one of those wires." How I wished that wand were magical. *Poof!*

"Yes, I can see that. *And?"*

"The third image is from today's mammogram. This is your incision from the lumpectomy, and this is the area where breast tissue was removed. That looks nice. Dr. Gallos did a wonderful job."

Hold the applause.

"What is that tiny white spot to the left of the incision?" I asked Dr. Newton. "It looks like it's in the same place as the photo with the wires that showed Dr. Gallos where she was supposed to cut. It's also on the first image from a year ago."

"Well, that's the area that concerns me . . ."

I butted in before she could complete her thought.

"Is that a speck of calcification? Did it get left behind? Why is it still there? Why wasn't it cut out?" I rambled.

The dialogue was over. I continued in monologue. "Now I remember. That was the shadow that didn't get biopsied back in January because during the procedure, the needle broke vessels in my breast and I started to bleed so badly. The radiologist had to withdraw the needle before he had the chance to take a sample of the calcification. He had to stop the procedure to address the bleeding."

Dr. Newton started flipping through the records in my file, trying to familiarize herself with my case history.

My panic found its escape through my mouth. My ranting continued. "I distinctly remember Dr. Gallos telling me that since that speck didn't get biopsied, she'd include it in the scoop of tissue she'd remove that contained the known cancerous tumor. The two spots were so close in proximity, it made sense to just cut it out."

I stopped to take a much-needed breath, and Dr. Newton jumped in. "I'd have to discuss those details with Dr. Gallos, Terri. It could be that it was either so close to the wire she didn't know it was there, or your bruise was obstructing it . . . there are any number of potential explanations."

"Or the radiologist who threaded the wires marking the area to cut didn't take a wide enough arc to include the whole field of calcifications!" I rebutted.

I had advanced from panic-mode to outrage. Dr. Newton had read all the books on how to diplomatically counter a ranting patient, choosing her words ever so carefully so as not to incriminate herself, her peers, or heaven forbid, the hospital that held her reserved parking space.

"I understand why you're upset, Terri. Unfortunately I don't have a lot of answers for you at this point, having just come into your case today. As things stand right now, though, what concerns me is that there is a 'dusting' of calcification surrounding the shadow in question. If I were you, I would have the area biopsied. Just to be sure."

"Oh my God. Are you kidding me? Another needle biopsy? We're going backward instead of forward! I thought I was done with this mess."

My head was pounding from trying to keep my temper in check. Deep down I knew that it was fear that fed my fire.

"This is a travesty. We found my cancer early. Stage I. Such a tiny tumor, it was, in my oncologist's words, 'Almost not a tumor at all.' I suffered through a needle biopsy, an MRI, an MRI biopsy, and a lumpectomy. I got zapped thirty-three times with radiation, and now I'm on a five-year course of medication. We have the technology to show itsy-bitsy microscopic specks on x-rays. We knew the calcification was there. It's not a *new* speck. It showed up on every photo. And now you're telling me to have another biopsy?"

Dr. Newton, still remarkably calm, answered, "I'm not telling you to have the biopsy. However, I think it would be in your best interest to do so. I'll show the images to Dr. Gallos, and we'll have two other radiologists review them, as well. We'll put our heads together and get back to you with our recommendation. Let's not get ahead of ourselves. It could be residual calcification from your incision. We don't know at this point. I know this is upsetting, Terri. I'll call you tomorrow."

"In all fairness, Dr. Newton, I know that you're just the messenger. You're new on my case, but if I have the biopsy and the result is positive, I may be looking at another surgery. I'm out of vacation time at work. I'll have to squeeze the procedure into this calendar year for insurance purposes. I'm cooking a bird in one week, and oh, let's not forget about Christmas four weeks after I get done washing the turkey platter! The thought of a second surgery is outrageous. What's that expression carpenters use . . . 'measure twice, cut once.'? We shouldn't even be *having* this conversation!"

"I do understand. But we need to keep this in perspective and gather all the facts before we jump to any conclusions. I'll call you tomorrow."

Linda stood quietly in the back of the room throughout my tirade. She knew her place. Technicians did not interject their thoughts or opinions, however expert they might be, while radiologists had the floor. She rubbed my shoulder while we walked back to the dressing area.

"Dr. Newton is good, Terri. Really good. She knows her stuff."

I shook my head, "Well, this mammogram was hardly a yawn fest, Linda. How did this happen? We all knew the spot was there."

"I know."

She was also careful not to point a speculative finger at who or where the weak link was in the chain of events that led to this apparent oversight. I had the distinct feeling, though, that she had an idea. The more Dr. Newton talked, the more the same radiologist's name popped up in areas that posed challenges throughout my treatment. Dr. Drake. His name, three times, where difficulties arose: the blown vessels during the initial needle biopsy, the injecting of the dye that never found the sentinel lymph node, and the threading of the guide-wires for Dr. Gallos to follow during my lumpectomy surgery. Coincidental? Perhaps.

"Do me a favor, Linda?"

"Name it."

"Please tell Dr. Newton that Dr. Drake is never to touch me or have any involvement in my case again. I'd like my request to be documented in writing in my case file."

"I'm guessing that's already been noted," Linda responded.

Yawn fest, my ass.

Chapter 38

I sat in my car in the hospital parking lot for a few minutes trying to process what had just happened.

A spot got left behind. Someone didn't do their job. Human error? I don't think so. Negligence. Pure negligence. Should I be looking for a lawyer?

It felt like the roller coaster car I'd been living in for the last year had finally jumped the tracks and was free-falling into a ravine. How would I explain this mess to my co-workers when I got back to the office? To my family? I felt like such an idiot to have assumed everyone would do their jobs and do them right.

I didn't know I was supposed to check everyone's work when they were finished. Was I supposed to ask the pathologist, "Are you sure your microscope was in focus when you read the biopsy sample?" The radiologist who set the wires, "Are you sure you outlined the surgical boundaries accurately?" The surgeon, "Are you sure you cut out the *entire* tumor?" If I was the victim of negligence, why did I feel like I was the one who screwed up?

I drove back to the office on auto-pilot. I was hoping to slide into my spot at the reception desk without too much notice. No such luck.

Helen was the first to ask, "Terri, you're back! How'd everything go?"

"Not as I'd expected."

"Oh no. What happened?"

"The mammogram showed a speck of calcification that apparently didn't get cut out during my surgery. It's not new calcification. It's old. For whatever reason, it seems to have gotten left behind. The radiologist thinks I should have another biopsy." My eyes were starting to well up with tears.

"Another biopsy? You're kidding me."

"I wish."

"How'd that happen?"

"Beats me. Someone dropped the ball, I guess. I can't believe I might be starting this whole process over again."

"Can they monitor the spot over the next few months to see if it gets bigger?"

"That's an option. But at some point, if they still think it should be biopsied, the procedure will cost me another six or seven grand out-of-pocket. If I have it done before the end of this calendar year, it won't cost me anything. I've met my insurance deductible and out-of-pocket max for the year, so now everything's covered at one hundred per cent."

"That's a lot of money. Sounds like a no-brainer. If you agree to the biopsy, it should be done now."

The switchboard kept interrupting us, forcing me to switch the tempo and tone of my voice back and forth from hard-rock to easy-listening.

"The timing of all of this couldn't be worse, Helen. I'm cooking for Thanksgiving in a week, then there's all the prep that comes with Christmas. What if I need more surgery? Recovery? When am I going to squeeze all of this in?"

"You're getting ahead of yourself. The biopsy may come back negative. What does Ludwig think you should do?"

"I haven't called him yet. Can you have someone cover the phones for a few more minutes? I'll try to get hold of him."

"Absolutely."

The first thing out of Ludwig's mouth was, "Time to find a lawyer." He was angry. Livid.

Dr. Newton didn't get back to me until early evening the following day. The consensus of Dr. Gallos and two other radiologists was that it would be in my best interest to have the calcification biopsied. "Just to be sure."

Joy to the world! Another intrusive procedure. End-of-the-year Christmas bonuses to all the White Coats!

Chapter 39

There was an opening on the biopsy calendar the next day. I verified that Dr. Drake was not to be assigned to the procedure, and I booked the appointment.

Gee, it's easier to schedule a biopsy than it is a haircut.

Having already experienced the procedure last January, I knew what to expect this time. I drove myself to the hospital, and I intended to drive myself back to the office afterward. I didn't care if I was bleeding out of every hole in my body, I was NOT going to take a full day off of work like the last time. A woman radiologist, Dr. Berger, and Linda, my favorite radiology tech, briefed me before the procedure. As bitter and skeptical as I had become with the entire medical industry, Dr. Berger seemed genuinely empathetic about my misfortunate of having to endure another biopsy.

She sounds sincere. Or maybe she just wants to win my affection; one of those "people-pleasers." Jury's still out on this one.

Linda shared the x-ray image with me and showed me precisely how she would guide Dr. Berger to insert the needle.

"This is the calcification. I'm taking Dr. Berger in through the side of your breast instead of the top. It's the shortest distance, and a straight and direct route."

"I don't care if she goes in through my nose, just as long as I don't erupt like last time. The bruise Dr. Drake gave me in January hung on for three-and-a-half months. I started setting an extra place at the dinner table for it."

"There you go again, cracking me up."

"It's nervous tension. Some people shake. I turn into Henny Youngman."

"Henny who?" Linda asked.

"The comedian. Played a violin? Famous for his one-liners? Never mind."

"Well, I don't foresee any bleeding or bruising going on this time, Terri. Dr. Berger is an amazing radiologist. We're going to take good care of you. You've got my word."

Is that enough? Your word? Can I have that in writing, please? Witnessed and sealed by a notary public. In triplicate.

Linda loaded Kenny G into the portable CD player and dimmed the lights, while another tech assisted me in climbing up the step ladder and onto the biopsy table. It took a good five to ten minutes to get me situated into the precise position necessary for Dr. Berger to have the best access to her target. The goal was to hit the bull's eye in one needle stick. Somewhere between climbing onto the table and listening to the hypnotic music oozing out of Kenny's alto sax, I converted my fear into faith, and I placed my entire wager on Dr. Berger.

Although my head was turned to the wall, I could hear the voices of at least four different women, all assisting in the procedure. Everyone had a task.

"There are so many chicks in this room, we could start a book club."

Linda's voice to the others: "She cracks jokes when she's nervous."

Linda's voice again, "Dr. Berger is about to get started, Terri. You're in perfect position right now. It's critical that you lie perfectly still from this point on. Laura will stand next to you in your line of vision. If you need us to stop or experience any pain, let her know right away. Do you have any questions before we get started?"

"Yeah. What rhymes with 'biopsy'? I'm thinking of writing a poem."

Chapter 40

The procedure was over before it started. No pain. No bruising. Needle in. Needle out.

I've said it before, I'll say it again; women doctors rock.

We finished with a final mammogram, standard procedure after a breast biopsy.

"Come look at these films, Terri. Dr. Berger did an amazing job."

"Amazing?" I asked. *She uses that word a lot.*

"This is your breast before the biopsy. See all these white dust-like particles? They're microscopic calcifications," Linda explained.

She pinned another film to the lit backdrop. "This is your breast after Dr. Berger's biopsy. Do you see how clean it looks?"

"Oh my God. All that white stuff is gone. It's like she took a vacuum cleaner and sucked it all out."

"That's what I said. Amazing."

"She did all that tidying up without breaking any blood vessels or causing any bruising."

"Yes, she did. I told you she did nice work." Linda sounded like a proud mama.

"I wish I had my gold stars along. I would so give Dr. Berger a giant gold star." *From here on out, women doctors only on the team roster. Males need not try out.*

"All the samples will go to pathology today. We should have your results in twenty-four hours. Either Dr. Berger or I will give you a call tomorrow."

"Thanks, Linda. You're pretty amazing yourself."

Back to the waiting game. It never gets any easier. Every wait in the last year of my treatment held its own tension and urgency. They couldn't be ranked or categorized by size, weight, or importance. Every one of them was heavy. And every one of them sucked. You'd think I would have gained a little grace over the year, but I didn't. Poor Ludwig knew what to expect; the Seven Dwarves all rolled into one wife: Grumpy, Jumpy, Cranky, Edgy, Snivelly, Whiney, and Little-Miss-Pain-in-the-Rumpus!

I prayed, but with more sincerity than the superficial bargaining I had done earlier. The closer I came to the reality that I could be standing on the front line battling another round of cancer, the more honest I became.

If I am meant to fight again, then please empower me with the grace, strength, attitude, and weapons that will be useful in my battle. Help me to be the example I would want my kids to follow when they encounter obstacles in their lives. Let my eyes, ears, and heart be open to Your unconditional love and guidance, and to the love that surrounds me in the faces of friends and family. Let "victim" never cross my lips. Only "chosen one." In your name, Thy will be done.

Linda called me at the office the following afternoon. "Negative."

Thy will be done.

Chapter 41

With no tangible game plan given to me by my doctors as to how to stay cancer-free, I decided to take matters into my own hands. Lacking a formal medical education, I designed my defense strategy in large part by calling upon my old friends Instinct and Common Sense. One of my sis's favorite quotes is one from W.L. Bateman: "If you keep on doing what you've always done, you'll keep on getting what you've always got." I was not going to let history repeat itself by "doing what I've always done." Even with one clean mammogram to my credit, I still felt like I had a neon pink target on my back. But I figured a moving target was harder to hit than one that stood still. So that's what I did. I started moving. Cancer couldn't find me if I just kept moving.

From the very first second of my diagnosis, I never quite bought into the explanation that "Sometimes cancer just happens." Horse cakes. Nothing just happens. There's always a cause and effect. Settling for an explanation like that meant not having to dig deeper for the real answers. Clearly, I didn't have a clue about the answers or potential causes of my cancer, and if the White Coats knew, they weren't spilling. But I wasn't going to live the rest of my life shrugging my shoulders, passively chalking up life's lumps as unexplained happenings. Figuring out how to dodge what I couldn't see became the challenge. Then it dawned on me: *Terri, don't waste your time trying to dodge what you can't see. Concentrate on what you CAN see!*

My diet. I could see what I was eating and drinking. When I finally took the time to get my magnifying glass and read the ingredient lists on the packages in my freezer and pantry, I was shocked and embarrassed by what I saw: Carcinogens, toxins, synthetics, and chemicals. Having just spent the better part of the past year turbo-blasting my body of cancer cells, the last thing I wanted was to re-contaminate my squeaky-clean, radiation-bathed system with junk. I read a lot about "clean eating" and the health benefits of a "plant-based diet" (gads—black beans, root vegetables . . . *kale*?). One book that I read used the rule of thumb, "If it has a face or a mother, don't eat it." Plants don't have faces *or* mothers, but most of what I ate did. The more I read on nutrition, the more I saw the correlation between quality of fuel and quality of performance. Fuel a machine with garbage and it'll perform like garbage. *Thank you, Common Sense.*

I needed to create an environment where healthy cells wouldn't be overtaken by wild, hard-partying, noxious cancer cells. I discovered entire Internet websites dedicated to targeting foods that are known to cause cancer in mice and other furry critters. Some of these foods are suspected of causing cancer in humans. There are plenty of nutritionists, holistic health practitioners, and scientists pointing accusing fingers at our country's food industry, holding them responsible for the steady swell of cancer. I wondered what role the FDA (Food and Drug Administration) really has in monitoring the safety of the foods that find their way to our supermarket shelves. Does the FDA have any interest in protecting America's consumers?

Let the buyer beware.

Grocery shopping became a literary experience, as I read every nutritional label on every package of food before tossing it into my shopping cart. I skipped past the total calories, fat, carbs, and protein chart, and I zeroed in on the ingredients. If I read a word I couldn't pronounce or find a picture of in my head, the item went back on the store shelf. No more pesticides, herbicides, sodium nitrites, nitrates, rBGH, MSG, BPA, caramel coloring, yellow dye #6, blue dye #3, red dye #3 or green dye #3. Who in their right mind would want to eat paint?! I especially turned a cold shoulder to artificial sweeteners such as aspartame, Sweet 'n Low, Splenda and Equal. There wasn't a single piece of literature I read that had anything positive to say about the short- or long-term effects on the human brain from these laboratory-bred, pink, yellow, and powder blue-packeted faux sugars. If it wasn't organic, it didn't come home with me. Most of my friends told me I was nuts. They said I couldn't prove that my food choices, past, present, or future, had anything to do with my getting cancer.

"Terri, that stuff on your hit list . . . it's in everything. You can't possibly escape all those toxins. What *are* you going to eat and drink? Pinecones and dandelion wine?"

I'd shoot back, "No, toxins and poisons are *not* in everything, and when *you* have to stuff one of your bra cups with a silicone cookie to fill the empty space, you might give more thought to what *you* eat and drink!"

That usually shut them up. I didn't care if they thought I was over-reacting or paranoid. Maybe I was both. But like my mom used to say, "It's no skin off my nose what they think, either way."

Unfortunately, I had a lifetime of not-so-enlightened-food-consumption to undo. I was born in 1958, which makes me a Baby Boomer. As a kid I subsisted on morning scoops of dry cereals like Trix (are for kids!), Lucky Charms (magically delicious) and Coco Puffs (I was coocoo for them.). We didn't have freshly-squeezed orange juice in our fridge. We got our morning kick by mixing a super-fine, pale orange-colored powder called Tang with water from the kitchen faucet. Heck, the astronauts drank Tang on their way to the moon. If it was good enough for them, I suppose it was good enough for me and my sisters. Right?

Lunchtime staples were pink (too pink) bologna or olive loaf on spongy white Wonder bread (as in, "I Wonder if this is really bread?"), canned Spaghettios, Beenie Weenie with a slice of Wonder bread to mop up the leftover juices, and fried Spam or liver sausage on toast (white, Wonder bread toast). Our brown sack lunches always included a snack bag of Geyser or Mrs. Howe's potato chips and either a Hostess Twinkie, Snowball, or cellophane sleeve of HoHos to glue it all together.

On the tails of that day filled with sodium, refined flour, and synthetic desserts came what was known as "supper." Some of my friends called the last meal of the day "dinner," but for my family, it was plain old supper. Oven-baked TV dinners bubbled in their metal compartmented trays. Soft, squishy wieners boiled in a stainless steel Revere Ware kettle on our avocado green stovetop. When the wiener water turned cloudy, the dogs were ready to meet either a single slice of Wonder bread as a wrapper, or if it was a good week, an official Wonder brand wiener bun. The traditional Friday night fare was Mrs. Paul's Fish Sticks (Fish? *Really?*), Tater Tots, and a bowl of canned creamed corn (all three of us girls hated that corn, and gulped back "the gags" to avoid getting thumped on our noggins or poked by Mom's fork for being picky eaters).

After we hand-washed and dried the dishes, we rounded out the night with a snack in front of "The Ed Sullivan Show" or "Leave it to Beaver." We heated and vigorously shook a flat pan of popcorn over the gas flame burner on the stove, waiting for the pan to erupt into a huge, silver foil beehive. Man, that Jiffy Pop was one cool invention! Or we sucked on Popsicles that stained our lips and tongues in freakishly bright shades of blue, red, orange, or green for the better part of a week.

That was what kids of the 50s and 60s ate. At least that's what we ate in my house. Our young bodies were toxic dumps. Chemical wastelands. My parents were both chain-smoking cigarette suckers, so their smoke was our smoke, too—in our house and in our car, nothing but second-hand smoke. It's a miracle any of us made it to puberty, much less adolescence.

That was my nutritional base. My teen and young adult years weren't much better. I take full credit for steadily contaminating my body with junk food, Coca Cola, deep-fried haystacks of shredded onions, breaded mozzarella sticks and chicken parts, fast food, frozen dinners, beef, pork, fatty bratwurst, and jumbo tubs of theatre popcorn dripping in motor oil. The list goes on. For most of those years I was lucky enough to be super-model thin, so the threat of gaining weight was never an issue. A blessed metabolism allowed me to eat anything I wanted and never gain a pound. I figured that meant I was healthy. I had no concept of the potential negative long-term effects of feasting on plate after plate of deep-fried pollution. Beyond the food pyramid, nutrition didn't seem to be a topic of interest to the news media either. Like thousands of lemmings, we followed the lively tunes and advertising jingles on our radios and TVs, luring us toward the latest, greatest, new and improved flavor of the day.

I can't help but wonder if the cumulative effect of my past eating habits was laying the foundation for my cancer. I'm no expert, but what if, just what if there is some truth to the theory that what we eat and drink does matter? What if we're our own worst enemy? What if *we* are the ones holding the smoking gun, and the cause of our own susceptibility to illness, disease, and yes, even cancer, is our own damned fault? Just what if?

Ludwig and I continued educating ourselves on clean eating, and gradually we integrated more ground-grown foods into our diets. It wasn't too hard to give up foods that had faces or mothers, because whatever junk those cows, pigs, or birds ate, we ate, too. *Yuk.* If they were injected with growth hormones or stimulants so they'd produce whiter milk, redder meat, juicier breasts, or so they'd drop eggs into their cardboard cartons at staccato speeds, then we were eating those chemicals, too. Even simple plants like wheat and corn have been genetically altered. Fruits and vegetables have been scientifically engineered and crossbred into plumcots, grapples, lematoes, pomatoes, broccoflower, rabbage. *Nectacotums? Now they've gone too far!*

At times it was a challenge to find foods in their purest forms. Sometimes what we threw together and liberally called a "meal" was far from mouth-watering. But we didn't give up or give in to our old habits. We scoured websites for palatable recipes. I wasn't beyond asking fellow shoppers at the farmers' markets and organic grocery stores, "I'm new at this. What do I do with this freaky little vegetable when I get it home?" Sometimes I got a facial response that implied I was the freaky little vegetable, but most times I got helpful advice. Imagination, letting go of traditional rules and methods of cooking that had been ingrained in me for 30-plus years, and gallons of organic salsa saw me through to some pretty interesting concoctions.

"So what's on the menu tonight, Terri?"

"How does Black Bean Sweet Potato Chili sound, oh lucky husband?"

"Have we had that yet?"

"Nope. But trust me, you're going to want it every night of the week, it smells so good!"

"Every night of the week?" Ludwig's eyebrows arched in bewilderment.

"Yup. I doubled the recipe. Belly-up to the trough, Sweet Potato! Get it while it's hot."

The kids thought we were a couple of hippies with our all-natural-this and our organic-that. One day Ellie and I were talking on the phone and she said, "Mom, what if you go to all the trouble of giving up grilled burgers and Friday fish fries, and eat nothing but that disgusting tofu and tree bark, and then you end up getting hit with cancer again anyway?"

"Well, I'm going to be damned mad, that's for sure. But I have to try. And I'll keep on trying until I get it right. Cancer doesn't just happen. I'll never accept that. And you shouldn't either."

If you keep on doing what you've always done, you'll keep on getting what you've always got. Memorize it, Ellie. You too, Karl.

Chapter 42

The elephant was back. It lumbered through every room of my house, leaving its dusty footprints and hot breath in every corner of my life. Like a child hiding behind tightly closed eyes, I pretended away the heft and smell of that old, wrinkled elephant. In the dark shelter behind the woven lattice of my fingers, I was able to ignore a lot of things—even the flag on my calendar reminding me it was time to schedule my next diagnostic mammogram. Aside from bumping into walls, living behind closed eyes had its benefits. Avoiding hard truths was one of them.

Seven months had passed since my last test, and the memory of that debacle is what had me so upset. I was afraid this new mammogram would reveal more clusters of microcalcifications, just like last time. Then I'd need another biopsy. Then I'd have to wait for the results of the biopsy. And what if the results came back positive this time? I'd need more surgery. Maybe a full mastectomy. Maybe this time I'd need chemo. I'd lose my hair. Sue. Nora. Cancer hit them twice. Why not me? What if my first cancer was just a warm-up for Round Two? What if this time I didn't survive? I felt the boney fingers of anxiety squeezing the breath out of me as July 3, 2012 came closer.

Each day the chorus of well-wishers who tried to ease my anxiety grew more irritating.

"Calm down, Terri. You'll be fine. I know it."

"You're getting worked up over nothing. Your mammogram is going to be perfectly clean."

"Trust me. You don't have cancer. You're fine."

"If anyone is cancer-free, it's you."

And my all-time favorite: "Think positive."

Good advice. I'll wear a smiley face pin on my lapel. That'll make a HUGE difference.

Why did everyone feel the need to predict my future or pretend that they could? As well- intentioned as their words of encouragement probably were, they sounded hollow, patronizing, and I felt were designed to comfort themselves more than to comfort me. What I needed from my friends was their quiet, compassionate acceptance of my fear. I needed them to simply ride the wave with me and keep me from drowning if I fell overboard.

My appointment was scheduled for 10:20 a.m., so I needed to take an hour or so off from work. I was a nervous wreck all morning, and while I prepared myself for the worst case scenario, a part of me still hoped, prayed, and pleaded with The Almighty for clean, spotless images. I wondered if I would ever feel completely free of the fear of a second cancer diagnosis. I felt like all the months I'd devoted to re-building my emotional, spiritual, and physical health were for naught. The confidence and faith I'd worked so hard to regain now bailed on me.

Maybe I'll cancel the appointment and go back to hiding behind closed eyes.

Marie covered the switchboard for me. "Good luck with your mammogram, Terri. Think positive!" *Grrrrr.*

"Thanks, Marie. If all goes well, I should be back within the hour."

I drove my old familiar route to the hospital. A cop was tucked away in his usual side-street hideout, waiting to make someone's day with a fat speeding ticket or fine for rolling a stop sign. I laughed out loud, and shouted through my closed driver-side window, "Cripes. Get a real job, Officer Krupke!" Then I gave him a toothy smile and a wave, laughing even harder, knowing in my heart it was fear that motivated my silly, bad-girl behavior.

The friendly volunteers with the ruby red smiles greeted me at the main desk and asked if I needed help or directions. I assured them I was familiar with the real estate. By the blank expressions on their faces, I surmised they didn't get the joke, so I back-pedaled and said, "Thanks anyway, ladies. I'm good."

I weaved my way through highly polished hallways to the Breast Care Center. My head was throbbing, and I felt a slight shortness of breath as I waited in the reception area for my name to be called. *Maybe I should have asked those ladies to direct me to the Intensive Cardiac Unit. I think I'm having a damn heart attack.*

"Hi, Terri. It's me again. Linda. Remember?"

"How could I forget? Are you stalking me?"

"Hardly. The sad truth is I don't have a life. That's why I'm here every time you come in!"

"Your loss, my gain. You know you're my favorite Radio Tech, right?"

"Thanks, Terri, I like you too. Back to business. How are you doing?"

Doing?

"Oh, I'm fine. Just looking forward to getting this whole thing over with. You might remember the scare we had seven months ago?"

"I'd like to take credit for remembering, but actually I read it in your chart before I came out to get you. That's not going to happen this time. You gotta think positive, Terri."

There it is again. Think positive. Linda . . . how could you?

The mammogram procedure was all too familiar—uncomfortable, but tolerable. I was praying I wouldn't pass out while my breast was still trapped in the waffle iron—that would be ugly—but I was one breath away from a full-blown anxiety attack. I kept hearing those words: "You've got cancer," over and over in my head.

"Okay, we're done here. Nice work. Have a seat in the waiting room. I'll be back in a few minutes with your preliminary results."

She looks so calm. I wonder if she practices in front of a mirror?

I obediently retreated to the waiting room and waited for the next 143 hours . . . with my eyes closed. *If I keep my eyes closed the cancer won't find me.*

Linda gently tapped me on the shoulder. "You taking a little nap, Terri?"

"Not napping. Hiding. I was hiding."

"Hiding? Not very well. I found you."

No kidding.

Linda continued, "From what I could see, your images looked great. Congratulations."

"Really? Are you sure?" Tears welled in my eyes.

"Nothing jumped out at me, but I don't make the final call. You know the drill. A radiologist will read the films, and then you'll get a letter in the mail with their analysis."

"I remember: the Waiting Game."

"A few days, tops. Do you have any questions?" Linda asked.

"Just one. Did you happen to see a slow-moving elephant looking for the nearest exit?"

"Elephant? Not quite sure what that's all about, but I'm happy to see you've still got your sense of humor."

That I do. But I don't have cancer.

EPILOGUE - You're More Prepared Than You Know

There's no preparation for hearing the words, "You've got cancer."

But I came to realize that I'd been preparing my whole life for what happened the second after hearing those words, and every second that followed. Without my even knowing it, everything I needed to battle and survive cancer was already securely zipped into the pockets of my backpack. I was more prepared than I knew.

My prayer pocket. It was stuffed full from every unexplained fever the kids sweated through as babies, every tense moment when Ellie stepped into a batter's box or up to a free throw line, every night I waited to hear Karl's key in the door after a night out with his buddies, and every time I willed the phone to ring on a stormy night to hear Ludwig's voice: "The plane just landed. I'm safe." For every pair of shoes I'd ever worn—as a mother, wife, daughter, sister, friend, bereavement companion—I'd collected hundreds of prayers. In my darkest hours of wondering if I'd live to see my kids graduate from college, or enjoy long, lazy days of retirement with Ludwig, it was

187

such a relief to dig into my pack and feel the soft, familiar edges of my prayers touch my fingertips.

My endurance pocket. It's the one that adds most of the weight to my pack. It's heavy because it carries layers upon layers of callous, scar tissue, and gallons of the blood, sweat, and tears that I've shed living out the many roles and expectations of womanhood. Whenever I felt the physical and mental fatigue from my treatment sapping me of my energy, I dipped into my endurance pool and I bathed myself in the knowledge that heck, if I could survive raising two kids without dropping them on their heads, managing a household without burning the place down, and still look dang rockin' gorgeous at 53 years old, I could survive anything. Even cancer. You bet that pocket is heavy.

My organization pocket. During the 12 years I stayed at home with the kids, I juggled athletic schedules, music lessons, doctor appointments, parent/teacher conferences, band concerts, pasta parties, and school dances. The time management, quick reflexes, and memory skills I developed during those years prepared me to handle the constant flow of paperwork and doctor appointments that come with cancer treatment. I called upon every method of filing and paper-pushing from my past to tackle the storm of medical and insurance statements that washed up on my doorstep nearly every day. Honestly, my "Cancer Binder" would (not could) win a Nobel Prize if one existed for such a creation. I could offer seminars for people who not only have cancer, but worse than that, also carry the "Don't-Know-How-To-Deal-With-Paperwork" gene. I believe anyone can be cured of that disorder with intense training in the proper use of page-protectors, index cards, colored stickers, tabs, highlighters, and of course, the implementation of the two-inch-thick, three-ring binder.

My help pocket. This was, and still is, the most difficult one for me to open. It's not that it has a stubborn zipper—it's more my unwillingness to grab hold of the tab and call upon the friends and family inside. I'd made a silent promise to myself that I was going to get through all the ups, downs, ins, and outs of cancer without asking anyone for help. But as tiny as the doctors said my tumor was, the lump it left in my road was massive. As hard as I tried to overpower the strength of that bully on my own, I couldn't.

The first time I broke down and poked only the tip of my finger into my help pocket, the wail of a baby suffering through teething let loose . . . then the sobbing of a teenager, broken-hearted from puppy love gone wrong . . . shrill screams came from a mother-to-be, going through labor and delivery. The most painful sound that escaped from the pocket was the silent sound of agony that comes after learning a loved one has died. The screams for help sounded so familiar. Every one of them was from me.

I punched my whole fist clear to the bottom of the pocket, hoping to quiet all that weakness and desperation, and that's where I found the cold teether that soothed my sore gums as a baby, the warm embraces and consoling voices, the washcloth that cooled my forehead during my hours of labor, a shot or two of whiskey, and a bubbling, fresh-out-of-the-oven Tater Tot casserole, prepared by neighbors upon hearing of Paula's death. Deep within that pocket were the friends and family who had seen me through so many of the painful events I'd already endured, from baby to adulthood, and I felt them stroking my angry, shaking fist until it relaxed. I was selfish to think my cancer was mine alone to fight. They wanted to pick up a sword and take their stab at the dragon, too! When I gave them their chance to help, I no longer felt the need to scream. I knew I wasn't alone in my battle. I knew they had my back.

My self-pity pocket. It's the prettiest, most accessible, and easiest to open of all the compartments in my backpack, but is the most useless pocket of all. It doesn't have a zipper or clasp to contain the beating of chests, complaining, and incessant whining that gets dumped there. On my "You've got cancer" day, the confusion, fear, anger, and despair I felt was unbearable—I cried most of the day and into the night. When I couldn't cry one more tear, I turned to my beautiful pocket, thinking I'd find a bit of comfort inside. I lifted the flap, and a vacuum sucked my hand deep into its darkness. The moaning and groaning was deafening: "Why me?" "What did I do to deserve this?" "Thanks a lot, God. Thanks for nothin'!" "You happy, Cancer? You found another life to ruin!" My voice. Not only the hysterical rantings from the day, but every blame-game and angry accusation I'd ever shouted, replayed in high-pitched definition. It was a loud and useless pocket, and there I was, wallowing in it up to my elbow.

While I'm not usually one to mope, I've been known to visit this pocket on occasion. Sometimes it feels good to stomp my feet, shake my fist, and blame someone else for the landmines in my life. It's a pocket that I should empty often. Life is hard enough without lugging around the extra weight of all that gloom and doom.

My faith pocket. The seams of this pocket are ready to burst from hundreds of beautiful memories. Faith brought Ludwig into my life when I thought I'd never find a companion to grow old with. It carried me through my pregnancies and the births of my beautiful, healthy daughter and son. Faith drove me to the hospital when Karl was five and wiped out on his rollerblades, breaking his chin open on the pavement . . . and again when he was eight and crashed and burned on his snow board, snapping his little collarbone in two. Ellie waited breathlessly to receive the acceptance letter from her first-choice university, and faith showed up in a big, white envelope with the word *"Yes!"* printed in red ink on the back. After my older sister Pauline died, faith dried my tears night after night as I cried myself to sleep. Faith persisted, and it woke me up every morning after, forcing me to leave the security of my down-covered cave and feel the warmth of the sun on my face. Faith never gives up.

While this should be the first pocket I go to for strength and compassion, it's usually the last one I pull from, after I've exhausted and emptied all the rest. For every time I've ignored my faith and tried to muscle my way through obstacles on my own, faith has stood silently waiting with patience and loyalty, ready to take my hand and guide me through my fears. Faith can't be seen—I suppose that's why I sometimes forget this pocket exists—but it's there. Although our course isn't always straight or free of lumps, faith's persistence always finds a passageway to hope when we give it a chance.

Cancer isn't the first lump I've ever stared down, and I'd bet my other breast that it won't be the last. Lumps come in all shapes and sizes—death of a loved one, unemployment, addiction, financial ruin, loneliness, fires, floods, and sometimes simply locking your keys in the car during a thunderstorm. I believe that we live our lives in constant preparation for things unseen. I can't predict what my next lump will be . . . heck, it might even be another bout with cancer . . . but whatever it is, everything I'll need to deal with it is securely zipped into the pockets of my backpack. I know that now. I'll be ready.

Acknowledgements

Words that live inside me have no shape or edges and care little about structure, tense or punctuation. They are happiest when they are free to wander aimlessly within the warmth and security of my heart and soul. Figuring out how to turn my internal words and memories into external words on a page was a challenge and remains a challenge. Stringing all those thoughts and words together into enough sentences to form a book was as bizarre a concept as the notion of how jumbo jets fly, how ships float, and how voices travel through the air in and out of tiny devices called cell phones. *Why don't all those voices bump into one another and end up in a heap of tangled gibberish?*

There's some truth to the adage: "It's not always what you know, but who you know, that matters." Thank you, to all my "whos" . . . you matter. You brought order to the chaos of my thoughts. You brought my book to life.

To my Kindle genius, Ludwig, thank you for figuring it all out! Your patience and quiet focus is so opposite my continuous frenzy-panic mode. I'd still be hammering away on a manual Underwood typewriter, or maybe an IBM Selectric, if I didn't have you to show me the way to technology. Your gentle tutoring has saved me from drop-kicking my laptop through our living room window dozens of times. If you had a nickel for every time I came to you in tears screaming that I was pretty sure I deleted my entire book, you'd have fur-lined bike shorts and a gold-plated BMW parked in our garage. You are my calm, my strength, my path to sanity. You will always be my Knight in Shining Armor.

Ellie, my beautiful daughter, thank you for sharing your heart in the Forward. Your reflection is honest and eloquent, two qualities I admire most in you. The quiet confidence you exude through your spoken and unspoken words, and through the life choices you've made as an independent, young woman, blanket those around you with warmth. Your sense of calm has sheltered me from many storms over the years. I am proud to be your Mom.

Thank you, Karl, for designing the front and back covers of my book. The miles and miles you and your Nikon traveled in search of my metaphorical cancer road, mean everything to me. Your instincts and perception of my cancer-journey led you to the perfect stretch of road. I am blessed to have a son with such deep insight.

Gail Grenier, my writing teacher and friend. Your expertise and honest, critical eye have guided me through so many multi-layered metaphors, tangled sentences, wrong word usages, run-on sentences, and fragments. You taught me it's okay to write long, as long as I write tight, and stuck with me every time I butchered the use of lay, laid, lain, lie, and lied. (I still don't know the difference.) Most of all, Gail, thank you for infusing me with the courage to believe that even though you are the teacher and I am the student, in the end it's still my story, and I get the final say! You are a heaven-sent mentor. And cheerleader. (That fragment's for you!)

Still too afraid to fly on my own when Gail's teaching schedule no longer coincided with my life schedule, I was fortunate to have another talented writing instructor enter my life. Cyndy Salamati, you met me and my book while I was writing the final chapters. A new set of eyes and perspective has been so helpful, especially as I laid (lay? lied? There it is again!) down my final words. Thank you for keeping me motivated and nudging me toward the finish line.

Special thanks to my fellow word-weavers from my writing class. I wrote most of this book in 1,000 word segments, and I read it to you during our class time, inviting you to share your critiques and impressions. You've been such a good sounding board. Some of your suggestions I implemented—some I "took under consideration." I encourage you all to step out of your comfort zone and share your creativity by submitting your work for publication. Believe with conviction that you are gifted and talented writers. There are critics who may not agree, but rejection letters fold into great paper airplanes. Send each one of them into the horizon and know that one day you *will* have the last laugh.

Beth Hoffmann, my proofreader/copy editor, thank you for dotting my i's and crossing my t's. The art of pure grammar has been pushed to the back row in the modern-day world of abbreviated texting and tweeting, and I applaud your commitment to sharing your technical skills with my readers. You are a diamond! (Confession: I broke down and took a few liberties with some of your corrections—I couldn't resist—call me a rebel.)

Special thanks to the dozens of unnamed friends, family, and co-workers that showed patience, tolerance, and encouragement as I sewed my story together, word by word, sentence by sentence. You saw me through many episodes of brain-freeze, brain-drain, writer's block, pessimism and procrastination, and you convinced me that moving forward, even if it was one baby word at a time, was better than not moving at all. I am so grateful you didn't allow me to stop before my dream of writing and self-publishing my story became a reality.

And finally, thank you, Pauline, my spirit sister. So many times I felt your energy coursing through my heart and out my fingers as I tapped letters into words on my laptop. My dream is to become the author you were meant to be.

Blessings to all of you, and all *you* dream to be.

Terri

Meet the Author

Terri and her husband, Ludwig, live in an empty nest in the village of Merton, a tiny suburb in southeast Wisconsin. Their children, Ellie and Karl, are finding their way as young adults in a wide-open world, and they bring reason, breath, and hope to each waking day. Terri enjoys writing essays and stories from her heart. *A Lump in the Road* marks her debut.

Contact Terri at: terrienghofer@aol.com

23224438R00121

Made in the USA
Charleston, SC
14 October 2013